DR. SEBI CURES BOOK

The Complete Guide to Naturally Detox your Body, Stop Disease, Cease Smoking, and Lose Weight with Dr. Sebis's Alkaline diet.

By

Rachel Voight

TABLE OF CONTENTS

INTRODUCTION

Research studies have shown that a diet based on plants can improve our health. In a 2015 study, a vegan diet resulted in more weight loss than other less restrictive diets. After six months on a vegan diet, participants lost up to 7.5% of their body weight.

Concerning appetite management, a study in 2016 of young male participants found that after consuming a meal of plants containing peas and beans, they feel more complete and happy than a meal containing meat. In a 2019 report, a plant-based diet could favorably alter the microbiome, contributing to a reduced risk of illness.

Likewise, a 2017 study showed that herbal diets could reduce by 40 percent the risk of coronary heart disease and by half the risk of developing metabolic syndrome and type 2 diabetes.

Dr. Sebi's diet allows people to consume whole foods and eliminates food processing. A 2017 study found that reducing processed food consumption in the United States would increase the general diet's nutritional quality. Dr. Sebi's diet does not contain enough essential nutrients not explicitly identified by the diet website. If a person consumes this diet, they can benefit from consulting a healthcare professional who can prescribe more supplements.

Following the diet of Dr. Sebi, a deficiency in vitamin B-12 can result. An individual can prevent this by eating vitamins and fortified foods. Vitamin B-12 is an important nutrient required for the health and the development of DNA in nerves and blood cells. Generally, the possibility of B-12 deficiency is presented for people adopting vegetarian diets and older adults. Doctors typically prescribe B-12 supplements for people who do not eat animal products.

B-12 deficiency signs include exhaustion, depression, and tingling in the hands and feet. There is also a chance of pernicious anemia that prevents the body from producing adequate red blood cells. Protein contributes to the brain's well-being, muscles, bones, hormones, and DNA in the diet. In compliance with current directives, women over 19 years of age are expected to have a daily intake of 46 g of protein, whereas men of the same age are expected to take 56 g.

Any of Dr. Sebi's diet foods contain protein. One hundred grams of oven-red chicken breast contains 16.79 g of nutrient, for comparison. However, Dr. Sebi's diet limits other plant protein sources, such as beans, lens, and soy. An individual will have to consume an extraordinarily large amount of the approved protein sources to satisfy daily needs.

Research indicates that it is important to eat a wide range of plant foods to consume adequate amino acids that constitute protein blocks. Omega-3 fatty acids are also essential for cell membrane components. Dr. Sebi's diet contains omega-3 plant sources, such as hemp and walnuts.

Anyone following Dr. Sebi's diet will benefit from a supplement of omega-3. Dr. Sebi's recipes also involve rare or proprietary botanical ingredients. An individual who does not adhere strictly to the diet, however, may easily adapt certain recipes to make nutritious, herbal food.

About Dr. Sebi's 'veggie-fuel' smoothie, try to leave off the date sugar, as, without it, the drink can be sweet enough. Sugar dates may be supplemented by maple syrup or cocoa sugar. Those who eat wheat or maize may prefer tortillas.

Scientific studies do not validate Dr. Sebi's diet. However, it can offer some of the advantages of other plant-based diets. Further intake of whole fruits and vegetables may have beneficial health effects. It can also help a person lose weight if that's an objective.

However, the limitations on Dr. Sebi's diet could pose risks. It is vital to ensure that the body is supplied with adequate nutrients, including vitamin B-12, if necessary. Some individuals may be more prone to the dangers of Dr. Sebi's diet. Among them are children, breastfeeding women, and older adults.

Diet advocates suggest costly items that are not validated by empirical evidence. More vegetable-based foods and any missing nutrients can be a better solution. It can be a good idea for a healthcare practitioner to perform research and consult before trying a new diet.

This GUIDE explores the composition and benefits of adopting Dr. Sebi's diet for revitalizing your body through a natural detoxification process.

Let's get started.

CHAPTER 1

WHO IS DR. SEBI?

Alfredo Bowman, known as Dr. Sebi, was a self-proclaimed Honduran herbalist. He was self-educated and had no formal physician training, according to his website. He was not a surgeon, nor did he hold a doctorate.

He immigrated to the United States and had multiple health problems, including diabetes, asthma, impotence, and obesity unsuccessfully treated. His website says he was cured by an herbalist in Mexico who inspired him to make his herbal blends, named Dr. Sebi's Cell Food.

According to the Health Line, he originally claimed that his herbs would treat chronic disorders like AIDS, sickle cell anemia, and lupus. But he was convicted without a license in 1987 for practicing medicine (although the jury acquitted him). Following another complaint by New York a few years later, Sebi decided to quit implying that his drugs could cure all illnesses.

Although controversial, Sebi's customer list reportedly included: John Travolta, Michael Jackson, and Steven Seagal. Sebi was arrested in 2016 for money laundering. During his incarceration in Honduras, he contracted pneumonia and died on his way to the hospital.

The man who worked on Nipsey Hussle, his documentary, was also murdered, while some took his death and Sebi's as proof of plotting shadow powers to suppress the truth about Sebi's remedies.

Sebi's key conviction assumes that alkaline foods and herbs (pH>7) are required to control the acid in our bodies, so preserving this alkaline state protects us from mucus buildup leading to disease. As our long-awaited Savior, alkaline coronation reveals a profound ignorance of the human body.

Sebi-African bio-minerals

Simply put, Sebi's Cell Food products are spices, algae, and algae known as African Bio-Mineral Balance products; a bottle of Bromide Plus capsules containing "Irish sea moss" and the bladder wrack is available for $30. Any of these ingredients may be related to allergies, intolerance, or medication. I don't know the big responsibility.

Many Sebi compounds are marketed as a detoxification solution, but we should know our body doesn't need daily detoxification. We are told the contaminants are still ambiguous and not well-defined, so we never saw the detox solutions we offer affect these disgusting boogeymen. "The gene resonates electrically in Africa."

Unfortunately, Sebi's health conviction went beyond conventional nonsense and race pseudoscience. Sebi also reported that African genes have high resonance and naturally "compliments [sic] the African gene structure." Genes are non-resonant.

You can wonder about your genetic heritage kits, telling you that your ancestors came from Ireland and Tunisia. Although their accuracy is at stake, they search for single-letter changes across your genome and compare your pattern with a reference community reporting itself in one region. Pure driving is the concept of genes vibrating at certain frequencies that decide your food needs.

The internet is full of self-trained gurus who profess to be every disease's only true cause and panacea. Unfortunately, true science slowly traces, painting the picture of a complex world in which different diseases have different causes, and therapies are imperfect, often having side effects.

CHAPTER 2

WHAT IS THE DR. SEBI DIET?

Sebi believed diseases are caused by mucus and body acidity and argued that diseases could not be found in an alkaline climate. This plan, which involves a strict diet and pricey supplements, claims to restore alkalinity AND detoxify the body.

The diet restricts animal products and concentrates on vegan food, but with much tighter laws. It limits seedless berries, for instance, and only allows Sebi's approved list of "natural growing grains."

Here's a short list of his diet guide's foods:

Vegetables: Amaranth greens, chayotes, avocado, cucumber, garbanzo beans, isots, dandelions greens, kale, lettuce (all but Iceberg), nopales, okra, olives, onions, mushrooms (all except shiitake), sea vegetables, squash, tomatoes.

Fruit: Apples, bananas, berries (all kinds of fruits), cantaloupes, elderberries cereals, currants, dates, figs, grapes of grapes, lime, oranges, peaches, pears, mangoes, melons feathers, pears, plums, soft gelatos, soursops (seeds), tamarind pears, raisins, soft gourd cocoa

Herbal teas: burdock, fennel, ginger, chamomile, fennel, raspberry, linden.

Plants: Amaranth, quinoa, rye, fonio, Kamut.

Nuts, seeds: raw sesame seeds, hemp seeds, raw sonic butter "tahini" walnuts, Brazilian nuts.

Oils: Olive oil (not cook pasta oil, sesame oil), coconut oil, hemp oil, avocado oil.

Basil, garlic, dill, orange, savory, leavened bread, sweet basil, achiote, cayenne, tarragon, thyme, onion powder, pure sea salt, habanero, sage, pure agave syrup, sugar date.

Sebi's diet guide also contains several other rules:

- You can only eat food listed in Sebi's Nutrition Guide
- One gallon of natural spring water must be drunk every day
- All animal products, including dairy, fish, and "hybrid" foods, are forbidden
- Alcohol is not allowed
- Sebi foods must be taken one hour before drugs
- You must avoid wheat and consume only the "natural-growing grains"
- No fruit (canned or seedless) are permitted
- Microwaves should be stopped

Is Dr. Sebi Diet sound?

The diet is highly deficient in protein: Sebi does not accept proteins, eggs, milk, or even soy from animals. It also limits the bulk of beans and legumes. Only some hemp seeds, walnuts, "natural growing grains," and brazil nuts have some protein in a diet. It can be very difficult to satisfy the dietary requirements of these products alone.

Protein is an essential component of all the cells in your body, and your body requires protein for tissue building and repair. Protein is a crucial component of the muscles, bones, skin, blood, and cartilage. Restricting macronutrients and major food groups can contribute to malnutrition.

While it promotes some fruits and vegetables, it oddly reduces a lot of items. For example, cherry or plum tomatoes are allowed, but there are no other kinds. Other types of items that it limits include lettuce and shiitake mushrooms, making the diet much harder to follow.

Sebi's main focus is on his complements that promise heavy "revitalize and engage intercellular advancement and "expedite the healing process. " Some packages cost up to $1,500 and do not mention nutrient and quantity data. That makes it hard to know how much you get from its proprietary mixtures and exactly what is in its supplements.

Sebi is not a physician in any form, and no evidence-based study is available to support his statements and recommendations. His extremely restrictive dietary recommendations promote eradicating major food groups, and macronutrients can have adverse health effects, leading to negative food ties. Knowing the facts and ensuring that science supports any diet you adopt is important to avoid a nutritional fog trap.

The plant-based diet is an alkaline diet designed to help cells repair through a combination of limited diet and supplements. The diet prescribes a strict veganism form, which is based on the assumption that all illnesses are related to a localized degradation of the mucus membranes present in the body. Based on this, the cause of sickness may be eliminated by maintaining an alkaline environment.

The diet also recommends taking supplements to Dr. Sebi Cell Food. Dietary rules:

1. It is not recommended if the food is not in the "Nutritional Guide."
2. Without trace, all Dr. Sebi items may be taken together.
3. Strict adherence to the "Nutritional Guide" (with additional products) offers the best outcomes for a disease reversal.
4. There is no consumption of agricultural products, hybrid food, dried fruit, seedless fruits, or alcohol.
5. According to Sebi, you "kill your food" with the microwave, stop it.

What does body alkalization mean?

The idea to control your body pH with the food you eat is an alkaline diet. As foods are used in our bodies, the belief is that waste may have a pH ranging between acidic and alkaline.

In different areas, the human body has different pH levels, with organs such as the more acidic stomach and more alkaline blood. Urines are a body product with a blood pH-management controller, directly influenced by the food we consume.

The wider category of "alkaline diets" focuses on the issue of metabolic waste, and Dr. Sebi's diets are among many and healthy to eat healthier plant foods. Still, there is no proof behind alkalization of the body, and research does not support his argument.

While the diet does make major claims, it cannot confirm it. It may lead to similar advantages as an alternative diet focused on plants where the benefits are better investigated, but protein sources tend not to have a strict dietary plan.

You may expect many benefits if you are considering trying a diet focused on plants. Here are some tips for starting your journey.

If you are interested, here is a complete list of Dr. Sebi's diet foods:

Plants

- Amaranth Greens
- Chayote (a Mexican squash)
- Kürbis
- Greens Dandelion
- Garbanzo beans
- Izote (cactus flowers/leaves)
- Mushrooms (but not shiitake)
- Nopales
- Okra
- Olives
- Onions
- Wonderful seafood
- Squash
- The peppers (only cherry or plum varieties)
- Tomatillos
- Toxins in zucchini
- Buggy Baby (verdolaga)

Fruit

- Apples
- Banana
- Beers
- Cantaloupe
- Cherries
- Dates

- Varieties of grapes
- Limes
- Mango
- Melons
- Orange
-
- Papayas
- Pear pinching
- Prunes
- Young coconut.

Oils

- Olive oil
- Coconut oil
- grapefruit Oil
- Sesame Oil
- Hempseed Oil

Noodles and seeds

- Hemp seeds
- Crude sesame seeds
- Raw Tahini
- Brazilian Nuts

Seasoning

- Basilique
- Bay Leaf
- Dill
- Savory
- Sweet Basil
- Tarragon
- Thyme
- Cayenne
- powdered Onion
- The Havanese
- Pure sea salt
- Pure agave syrup
- Saccharose Date

Teas

- The Kurds
- Chamomile
- Elderberry
- Fennel
- Raspberry

CHAPTER 3

THE ACIDITY OF
THE HUMAN BODY

Acidity Causes Damage To The Pancreas

Teachers use litmus paper tests in schools around the USA to prove that pH varies between acidity and alkalinity. However, is the definition of acidity and alkalinity relevant to everyday life? Yes, because every component of the human body has a survival pH. Therefore, people must promote the right pH in their bodies.

Scientists have established a calculation of acidity or alkalinity in various mineral solutions with a pH scale of 0 to 14. Any acidic solution that has a pH below 7.0 is acidic with the highest pH of acidity. Any solution with a pH above 7.0 is alkaline, with an alkaline pH 14.

When it's healthy, the human body maintains a slightly alkaline balance. Our blood pH is 7.4. If a person's blood pH drops to 7.0, a massive organ failure kills him or her. Organs like the heart, lungs, and brain need a steady blood pH of 7.4.

Therefore, the human body actively works to maintain the right pH, as every cell in the human body lives, breathes, and waste occurs, and these waste products are typically acidic.

Through many ways, the body may become too dangerously acidic if the body obtains too much acidic food, if cells contain too much acidic waste, or if these acids cannot be eliminated or neutralized by the body. If the acids cannot be neutralized or destroyed, the cells practically bathe in their waste. This disease is known as acidosis or excess acidity.

Acidosis erodes and eats in the heart membranes, artery, and vein cells in a way that acid slowly passes through some of the world's toughest materials, such as marble or metal. Over acidity is responsible for many diseases and premature aging by the gradual erosion and degradation of the body's cells.

Acidity and the pancreas

Certain body parts are more alkaline than others, of course. Highly alkaline glands such as the liver and pancreas are the most vulnerable to acidic damage. The pancreatic juice has a 7.8 to 8.0 pH.

The pH of the liver bile is from 7.5 to 8.8. But as the body's acidity increases, all pancreatic and bile juices become more acidic. Acidosis is the destructive, irritating, and inflammatory causes of bile and acidic pancreatic juices, stones, ulcers, and cancer of the pancreas and liver tissues.

Overly acidic bile also causes a reflux or bile backflow into the pancreas, the gut, stomach, and esophagus. Bile reflux is also associated with the duodenum and stomach, contributing to inflammation, ulcers, and cancer. Acid reflux and bile reflux frequently occur together, inflaming the esophagus and raising the esophageal cancer potentials.

Another concern with high overall acid toxicity or when the bile is in the pancreas is bile pancreas reflux. This bile backup can cause acute pancreatitis and worsen chronic pancreatitis problems. Acidic bile is also considered an essential factor in gallbladder stone production. Blocking the pancreas and bile ducts can cause substantial pancreatic damage and hepatic damage.

To make sufficiently alkaline pancreatic juice, minerals and bicarbonates are hard for pancreatic cells to gain when blood becomes too acidic. Several problems arise without alkaline pancreatic juice, such as:

- Less pancreatic enzymes cause indigestion of duodenum,
- Decreased protease inhibitor activity (the special enzymes that suppress protease from the digestion of its pancreas within the own pancreatic duct). Pancreatitis inflammation begins when the protease digests its pancreatic cells,
- Increased calcium pancreas that helps irritate pancreas stones,
- Decreased pancreatic juice anti-microbial properties,
- Spasm and the resulting Oddi sphincter blockage. This blockage increases the pancreatic pressure, which starts the digestion of pancreatic cells by trapped digestive enzymes. This causes discomfort, inflammation, and can cause the pancreas to die.

Healthy pancreas food, minerals:

Our current diet is naturally acidic and changes the body's pH balance to an acidic state known as metabolic acidosis.

Metabolic acidosis becomes more common as natural alkaline foods, such as fresh vegetables, move away from the normal US diet.

In acid-producing foods such as meat, most dairy products, white meals, sugar, alcohol, refined vegetable oils, soft drinks, and coffee, the body becomes acidic. Stress, sedentary living environments, smoking, free radicals, chronic inflammation, and infection often cause acidity in the body.

With an increased frequency of over-acidity, the condition is considered a dangerous illness that weakens the whole body. The body must extract alkaline minerals from key tissues, bones, and muscles to neutralize and disposing of high acidities.

These minerals have good health qualities, including calcium, magnesium, sodium, and potassium. When the pancreas leaks these vital minerals and bicarbonates, the pancreas is irritated, causing inflammation and cancer.

More minerals and bicarbonates need to be included in the diet to avoid over-acidity of the body. These minerals and bicarbonates are derived through the treatment of food and mineral water.

The way we eat today is completely different from our ancestors' diet and eating habits. Technology and its growth have changed all facets of our lives, including what we eat. Fast food is the norm in the busy world in which we work. Taking out food, cooking quickly for the packaged food we purchase in our supermarkets, and eating habits, such as eating while watching TV, are entirely the opposite of the lifestyle adopted by our ancestors.

The effect is less fruit and vegetables consumed, and at the same time, more processed products, milk products, and animal meat protein consumed. We compensate for what we consume with crash diets and low carbohydrate diets of high protein.

We wonder then, why in our lives, diseases such as heart conditions, various allergies, and bone diseases, which were not so common years ago, have become a reality. Doctors, nutritionists, and dieticians believe that what you eat affects your body and can be correlated with particular diseases such as those listed above.

Food influences the metabolism of our bodies and how it works every day. False foods will harm the body, causing health problems due to imbalance in the body. Thus, by changing our habits on what we eat, these health problems can be cured or ideally avoided.

CHAPTER 4

ALKALINE AND ACID BALANCE AND YOUR ENERGY LEVELS

All foods affect body acid/alkaline levels. Acids must be balanced to maintain good health. The body should be slightly alkaline for strength, endurance, and energy. An alkaline diet revitalizes and promotes natural health.

The term pH is "Potential of Hydrogen," calculating a solution's relative acidity or alkalinity. The pH level shows the body's acid/alkaline balance and tells the individual's health. The pH scale runs from 0-14. Zero is completely acidic and 14 alkaline. The mid-scale, seven, is neutral. Quality water has a pH of seven.

Very rarely is an individual too alkaline. It's more common in someone who eats little to no protein. However, for the vast majority, the problem is more acidic. Blood should be slightly alkaline (7.34- 7.45). This range means disease, under 7.0 pH is acidic. Over 7.0 pH is alkaline.

One must be careful not to develop an acidic pH balance due to eating so many proteins and grains. Too much stress can cause an acidic pH. Too many body toxins that rob cells of oxygen and nutrients may also create an acidic balance.

Acidic equilibrium effects:

- Body capacity to consume minerals and nutrients is jeopardized.
- Radical damage is heightened.
- Diminishes mental clarity.
- Physical energy diminishes.
- Insomnia and disturbed sleep cycles are common.
- Immune system impairment when helpful intestinal bacteria die.
- Colds, infections, and flu are common.

Alkaline foods typically include most apples, green vegetables, peas, beans, lentils, herbs, seasonings, seeds, and nuts.

Acid-forming foods include beef, fish, poultry, eggs, and legumes.

Drink eight-10 glasses of water a day.

Your emotional condition is also a significant health factor and can influence your pH. Meditation, tai chi, reflexology, massage, acupuncture, calming touch, relaxing music, and yoga are practices that buffer everyday acids and encourage an alkaline body.

But how can you control your pH to preserve alkalinity?

First, you buy pH paper in the drug store. First, select your saliva or urine, and extract either sample. Place the pH paper in contact with the specimen you selected and immediately compare the paper's color to the color code on the pH dispenser.

For an accurate reading of your health status, it is recommended that pH levels be reported for 30 days, three times a day, morning, afternoon, and night. Every day conduct the test simultaneously.

Cellfood/Oxygen Therapy

The culmination of 42 years of study is made of the finest plant substances, capable of maintaining the powerful elements in a complete solution, supplying them to each cell in the human body. This miraculous formula promotes and improves biochemical, nutritional activities and gives our diet what modern life and technology have taken away.

Cellfood contains enzymes, 78 trace minerals, 34 electrolytes, 17 amino acids, and nascent oxygen and hydrogen as products—all naturally occurring substances and important to the body's many biochemical functions, in a form that is easily absorbed by the body's cells. The body mistakes it for its fluids, absorbing it quickly and easily.

Cellfood provides the body with an abundance of oxygen and is considered one of the simplest ways of oxygen therapy. NucellCanada also supplies Master Detox, another substance that supplies oxygen at the cellular level, and Miracle Growth Factors, which is IGF-1, the essential nutrient that someone of any age can take.

It improves athletic prowess and sexual drive. Ocean Wonder Kelp for the proper functioning of thyroids and also provides oxygen. Cellfood anti-aging DNA/RNA is immune-improving, tissue-supporting.

Foot patches to eliminate harmful metals from the body. Stick patches on your foot to detoxify when you're sleeping. The body quickly absorbs Cellfood multi-vitamins as it's spay.

Gastric hyperacidity is a common medical disorder. Moreover, metabolic acidosis is the cause of all diseases as it is directly linked to multiple kidney disorders, diabetes, ulcers, and many other internal diseases. Hence the alkaline diet aims to normalize the pH and help people lose weight, not by a calorie deficit, but by replacing certain other acidic foods with alkaline foods.

An alkaline diet is a modern diet born from people's desire/need to manage gastric hyperacidity and avoid or delay as many acidosis-induced problems.

Alkaline diet strategy includes the development as follows:

A. 75% alkaline foods with a pH above 7.4, as close to eight; and
B. 25% acidic foods.

What's the difference between acidic and alkaline foods?

Normally, the internal pH (blood) is 7.38-7, 52. The pH mustn't drop below 7, as this can cause grade IV coma and patient death. The blood also doesn't have to have a very simple character, but just slightly alkaline. Otherwise, the possibility of involuntary muscle contractions is highly strong and painful.

What foods are alkaline, acidic?

In the alkaline diet group, we have:

A. Cheese, avocado cucumbers and lettuce, and all chlorophyll-rich vegetables;
B. Soy milk, lemon, millet, coconut, beans, and buckwheat;

C. Sea buckthorn's; and

D. Some cold-pressed oil;

Alkaline water is key to diet!

It is recommended that those who cannot achieve the prescribed percentage of diet (25% acidic and 75% alkaline foods) recommend substitute beverages with alkaline water.

Any water with pH above 7.7 is considered alkaline water and can be ingested in large amounts. The risk of increasing blood pH to vital values is very low; 2.5-3 liters of alkaline water a day can help preserve optimum health and help detoxify the body and clean, free radicals.

Smoking is forbidden!

Smoking is a practice that increases the body's acidity, which occurs when we drink alcohol. It is also recommended that these behaviors be reduced or omitted from everyday life so that the body has every chance to stay safe and clean. Smoking is strictly forbidden in alkaline diets.

Did you know that acid is the typical Western diet? This means that our foods cause a phenomenal blood imbalance, and did you know it could be extremely harmful to your health?

As you might know, the body is made up of 70% water. Hydrogen potential(pH) is an acidity or alkalinity measurement of the solution. The higher the pH, the more alkaline and oxygen are the richest fluid. The lower the pH, the less acidic and oxygen the fluid is.

However, when our diets are rich in acid-forming foods our diets lack enough alkaline material to make up for it, the acid begins to build up in our cells, causing them to be deprived of oxygen and die. If our body does not have the ideal pH, then vitamins and minerals cannot cure themselves or assimilate effectively. The pH levels affect everything, and therefore, alkaline pH balance needs to be maintained most of the time.

Test your pH levels by putting your urine in pH bands you can buy online or in health food stores. We advise you to test your levels more than once a day and record your readings for several weeks to ensure that your pH level is accurately reflected.

Your intake of healthy green vegetables, salads, sprouts, and fruit has to be increased if your pH levels fall below 7.0 most of the day. Raw food is better because it is filled with heat-destroying vitamins, minerals, and enzymes.

Acidic pH levels, some of which are listed below, can cause many health problems:

- Weight gain, obesity, and diabetes
- Immune deficiency
- Hormonal problems
- Slow digestion and treatment
- Bad hair, skin, clots
- Lack of energy and fatigue
- There are dying muscles, cramps, and spasms.
- Allergies, infections, and ulcers
- Depressing trends

The list goes on.

The list of health complaints may seem far too familiar, but it is important to know, and relatively easily, that the ideal pH level can be achieved. Cut down on dairy, meat, pasta, bread, rice, tea, coffee, and alcohol (all acidic foods) and increase your consumption of fresh raw fruit and vegetables (alkalizing foods).

Try dietary supplements of 60 percent alkaline food, up to 40 percent (maximum) acidic foods. We recommend many raw fruits and vegetables as snacks, as they are alkaline and help you lose weight, regain energy, and are healthy and delicious!

CHAPTER 5

REASONS TO GO ALKALINE AND AVOID ACIDS

The body is a wonderful tool, and its myriad processes and systems interlock to create a streamlined machine that works smoothly. As with all machines, however, the body needs the correct fuel to function correctly, and the waste products generated through the combustion of this fuel are flushed out without any problems.

The body might be perfectly balanced once, and perhaps humanity once lived in a perfectly balanced world, but we have become unbalanced over the millennia; both our diets and our ecosystem are overwhelmed with acids and acid waste—the problems associated with acidification range from fatigue, arthritis, depression, and cancer.

Although not much can be done on an individual scale in terms of global pollution level, we can control our diets and what we allow in our bodies.

It can appear as if following an alkaline diet requires a lot of effort and energy, but the benefits of going and remaining alkaline are far beyond the drawbacks. There are dozens of reasons to start an alkaline diet, and a book would take to list all but the top seven reasons to go alkaline and prevent acids are listed below.

1.) Weight Loss

The average Western diet and lifestyle consist of many acid-producing substances (refined meals, sugars, meat, and dairy products) and habits (smoking, consumption of alcohol, and prescribed pharmaceuticals) so that our bodies are flooded with acid waste.

One of the body's automatic defensive mechanisms is to make fat cells, to protect our delicate bodies against these excess acids. The function of fat cells is to shut these acid wastes away from our bodies and store them in less important parts of the body, but while there is an excess of acid within the body, the fat cells stick to their bodies defensively.

2.) Improved Energy

The more acids that form inside the body, the less efficient the body's natural equilibrium systems and the higher the body acid level. And the higher the levels of acids, the higher the levels of alkaline minerals (magnesium, calcium, phosphates, etc.) in the bones, tissues, and muscles are removed to ensure that blood maintains the alkaline levels needed to work in the body. If the efficient metabolism of these types of alkaline minerals is removed, it causes slowdown and fatigue.

3.) Allergy Relief

Acidic environments override the immune system and encourage the immune system into the so-called "response mode," which leads to an incredibly greater body's sensitivity to all kinds of things; pollens, chemicals, and so forth.

We know that this sensitivity is increased as allergies. Some of the other approaches the body can use soreness, swelling, eczema, and excess mucus to handle excess toxins and acidic waste are allergies-related. Once excess acids are removed, allergies and related symptoms disappear.

4.) Reverse the aging process

The aging is caused by acid waste accumulation and resulting body function disintegration. Acidosis occurs when the body is too acidic. The stress of oxidation systems and the collapse of lipids is simply acidosis. Free radicals are released into the bloodstream when this happens.

Cells attacking cell walls and membranes are free radicals; cell walls and membranes are killing before cells are torn. The visible result is discoloration, poor vision, aging, memory impairment, fatigue, and hormone dysfunction. By removing these acids, you can prevent further damage to your cells and reverse the break-up process.

5.) Oxidation

One of the side effects of the build-up of acid waste is that body cells do not receive sufficient oxygen, causing the cell to slow down in its myriad functions. Like the body itself, without enough oxygen, cells can die. By removing the acids built in your body, you can originate your blood by changing your diet and drinking alkaline water.

6.) Reduction of Blood Pressure

If a body is overly acidic, cells slow down (see #5), and the heart has to work harder to offset its leniency causing high blood pressure. Another side effect of high acidity is the increase of plaque in the arteries and a decline in blood vessel diameters, leading to higher blood pressure. You can improve your cell function by removing acid waste and remove some of your heart pressure.

7.) Decrease opportunities for the development of degenerative diseases

Increasing body acid waste (e.g., acidosis) has been the fundamental cause of almost all known diseases of degeneration, including diabetes, obesity, hepatitis, renal diseases, cardiovascular diseases, neurological conditions, premature aging, hormone imbalances, osteoporosis, and many other cancers.

In acidic environments, degenerative diseases thrive so that they are deprived of their ability to increase or even hold by removing their favorite environment.

What can you do?

If you want to solve any potential health problems, you can take one step right now to engage in an alkaline diet. You can get rid of acidic waste accumulation and turn the hands of time by choosing to eat alkaline (salads, fresh and raw vegetables, alkaline fruits, seeds, nuts) and drinking alkaline water for years.

CHAPTER 6

WHY ALKALINE IS ESSENTIAL TO YOUR DIET

Our body's fundamental biology tells us that a certain balance exists between alkaline and acid rations that our bodies need to be healthy. This ratio is calculated by the pH scale, with a pH of less than seven acidic, and seven alkaline.

When you eat high-acidic foods, the body's pH level is disrupted, shifting to an acidic pH. Fine sugars such as candy and some beverages, meat, and products made from meat, processed food, and condiments are examples of foods in this group.

The pH level in the blood is assessed. High levels of acid measured in the blood are a common factor for these diseases. Health experts and professionals from the sector agree that this high level of acid causes severe illnesses, even deaths, that we are suffering from today.

The opposite of and cure for acid are alkaline. Its key role in the body is to reverse and annul the harmful effect on our acid bodies. If the food we digest doesn't refill alkaline levels, it decreases to too low to counter acid.

How to get a balanced pH

The simplistic method of restoring the pH level in the body is to eat alkaline foods. This counteracts the harmful effects of high acidity as it travels through the body, damages organs, and kills soft tissue. Blood flows across the body, and the damage from elevated pH levels can also enter all areas of the body.

It is a simple and easy way to decide whether your body's pH balance is disrupted with strips calculating the pH level. Buy these measurement strips in your nearest drugstore or in shops that sell medical supplies. The pH level can be measured with strips that sample saliva or urine. The distinction between the two strip forms is:

- Saliva is measured - Acid output is measured. The normal dimensions are 6.5-7.5.
- Urine – Excess acid is excreted with those strips and weighed with them. Normally 6.0-6.5 in the early morning and 6.5-7.0 in the evening.

Too much acid endangers the body.

High acid levels or acidosis may cause various diseases. The basic symptoms caused by acidosis are:

- Cautionary headaches,
- Daily flu or colds, and
- Tiredness.

Diseases that may be due to acidosis are:

- Acne
- Bronchitis

- Depression
- Arthritis
- Dry skin
- Heart Complaints
- Hyper Acidity
- Infections
- Obesity
- Ulcers

Depleted alkaline levels cannot activate the negative and harmful effects of high acid levels as described before. Return the pH levels to normal by consuming the right foods; this raises the body's alkaline levels to normal levels.

Like processed foods, food containing additives should be excluded or consumed in limited quantities from your diet. Alcoholic drinks, milk products, beef, and meat products are other foods that are high in acidic levels. On the other side, fresh fruit and vegetables will replenish the body's alkaline levels. Fruits like lemons and oranges are naturally acidic but alkaline when digested.

The perfect diet consists of 75 percent of alkaline foods. A strong army has a stronger chance than a poor army for victory. Give your body the best opportunity to combat acid by increasing the alkaline level with the food you consume.

CHAPTER 7

ALKALINITY AS
THE SWEET LIFE

The alkalinity concept is often confused with the pH of the body. pH refers to the entire measuring scale from extremely sweet (0) to extremely sweet or basic (14) chemicals, with (7) being the midpoint known as neutral.

Think about the extremes of hot and cold water. The mixture of equal amounts of hot and cold water gives us an exactly mid-two hot extremes temperature. The equal mixing of acids and bases gives you a neutral pH that is neither acidic nor alkaline.

I think that misunderstanding generally occurs because the word alkaline's normal use is frequently equated to conditions larger than seven. Alkalinity refers only to the scale portion of 7-14.

The ideal condition of our bodies is 7.4 pH. Because we now know that our bodies work perfectly when they are only slightly alkaline, our bodily pH balance within this range is helpful. The final point is that all research shows that disease, including cancers, flourishes in an acidic environment.

Most health authorities say that the body's long-term excessive acidity effectively decreases our immune system's efficacy and usually contributes to chronic inflammation and disease.

Where can I begin to protect my health?

An excellent and economical way to show fast pH levels is to purchase ordinary litmus paper from most healthcare stores. A paper scale usually comes with the product that defines the true pH of saliva or urine by color codes. Insert your tongue, or urine, preferably on waking, with a small strip of paper.

The saliva pH levels are normally 7 or 7.5. The higher the alkaline, the lower the acid. You can search for alkaline or acid-specific foods to correct your levels once you have found out that you need to change your pH. These can be found readily on the web (Google + alkaline or acid foods), and you can also print out handy charts for your shopping trip.

The body consists of 70% water. Blood is the most vital fluid in your body. Then we can logically conclude that most of the blood is water. To function optimally, all your muscles, skin, and vital organs need massive amounts of water.

Water is the vehicle that transports oxygen to your cells. It eliminates waste and supplies energy. Adequate pH tested water supplies are essential for optimum health levels. You can increase the overall alkalinity by adding lemon juice or some other alkaline fruit.

With just a bit of research, you will find supplements that you can use every day to increase your alkaline and acid levels as your specific needs dictate. To keep your alkalinity constantly up, you may find specific things you will want to stop using and things you have to start using regularly.

What's to be avoided?

Typically, artificial sweeteners are very acidic and have negative effects on your nerve and digestive systems. There was a mistake (Sucralose, Nutrasweet, saccharin). Besides, some of these sweeteners have been associated with cancer.

Most of these red meats are extremely acidic and have really low water content. Stay away from red meats. Better to replace chicken, turkey, and fish with the protein we need.

Reduce the supply of processed and refined foods like a meal, preservatives, and coloring food. These foods are known to leave the body with acid residues. Besides, they are stored in the fat cells.

Stay away from foods that are fatty and fried, they also increase acid levels.

Alcohol increases our body's acid levels and should be avoided. It also significantly increases blood acid levels. Make alkaline water levels an alternative to alcohol; do not forget to add lemon.

Stress is a big blame. It increases acid and blood pressure as well as adrenaline in the bloodstream. It also causes the stomach to produce higher acid levels. You should counter with exercise the effects of stress; it increases alkalinity.

The optimization of alkalinity levels is imperative for good health. Diagnosis and treatment of pH are relatively simple and cost-effective for all. Your factor of sweetness is up to you. Don't expect your doctor to tell you this a crucial problem. Be hands-on of your own health.

CHAPTER 8

THE ALKALINE DIET PROS AND CONS

A balanced diet starts with an active lifestyle. Your workout and diet ultimately decide how you feel. Of course, there are limitless food plans, and one of them is the alkaline diet. Is it working?

What are the benefits and disadvantages?

Within this chapter, we will attempt to make some of these things clearer.

The basics: The alkaline diet has been around for a while now, but Victoria Beckham tweeted about it.

The diet is easy–eat foods that encourage alkaline, and diseases can be prevented! So the diet is based primarily on consuming nutritious things like fruits and vegetables, and some nuts, seeds, and lentils are also available.

Alternatively, you have to leave much of the food, including grains, meat, and milk, behind. Neither caffeine nor alcohol is permitted. You can't have any kind of food that is packaged or processed.

Pros at a glance:

First, with alkaline diets, you lose weight, so that's not disputed. Essentially, you remove the fats and other kinds of unhealthy foods, and the daily intake of calories will decrease. This is a balanced diet, and it is, in a way, healthier than the other fad diets. Thirdly, the alkaline diet does not require a lot of cooking, and you can handle this diet if you are a lazy chef.

On the flip side: Ok, the alkaline diet doesn't work as it says. Our body can regulate the pH level, and the food we consume has minimal impact. As such, you don't get the things others say exactly. There is also very little study on this diet, and thus no statements connected with it can be confirmed. The rules and meal plans for some people can be confusing, as different web tools can say different things.

What's a better choice?

The aim is to focus on a healthy diet. If you can follow the alkaline diet to the bone, you'll probably see some amazing results, but most people won't. Firstly, you must keep an eye on what you eat, and if you are a student, that can be difficult to control if you snack. The list of don'ts is also immense.

One smart option is to use alkaline water, which has the same benefits and can be a perfect substitute for standard water filters. Improved vitamin water has incorporated electrolytes, along with body-friendly calcium, potassium, and magnesium. Of course, it can't substitute the diet, but it's the best you can if you have no other choice.

Alkaline Diet Chart

The theory of an alkaline diet relies on the assumption that when we consume food, after digestion, either acid or alkaline bases are released to our systems. For example, acid is produced in foods like meats, poultry, milk products, grains, and salt.

The basis of fresh fruit and berries, legumes, nuts, and tuberous berries like potatoes is alkaline. Today, most contemporary physicians promote fresh fruit and vegetable intake, but most do not believe in acid and alkaline diet basics.

Many people believe that diets dependent on acid cause health issues such as fatigue, ovarian cysts, nervousness and irritability, chronic illnesses, such as colds, excessive mucous and nasal irritation, and a general lack of strength.

Some people assume that an acidic diet can cause cardiovascular harm, weight gain, obesity; diabetes; a weakened immune system; kidney stones; osteoporosis, premature aging, and slow digestion.

Alkaline diet supporters believe it maintains the body's normal pH balance between 7.35 and 7.45. Since our body's pH is slightly alkaline, our diet should be slightly alkaline, ranging from 7.36 to 7.44.

This balance tends to be upset by an unbalanced diet high in acidic foods such as animal protein, caffeine, sugar, and processed foods. It can make people susceptible to chronic and degenerative diseases by depleting alkaline mineral products such as sodium, potassium, magnesium, and calcium.

The internal chemical balance of our kidneys, lungs, intestines, and skin is largely controlled. To carry out the functions necessary, our body must have a proper pH. Measurement of the acidity or alkalinity of a substance is called pH.

Adequate alkaline reserves for optimal pH adaptation are required. To achieve pH-buffering, the body needs water, oxygen, and acid-buffering minerals while rapidly removing waste products.

The excessive acidification of the body is the cause of all diseases. Soda is probably the most acidic food people eat at 2.5 pH. Soda is 50 thousand times more acidic than neutral water and consumes a glass of soda for 32 glasses of neutral water.

The body should neutralize acids and toxins from the blood, lymph, and tissue while also strengthening the immune and organ system the sup of nutrients and alkaline food and water.

Most fruits and vegetables contain greater quantities of alkaline elements than other foodstuffs. The more green foods the diet consumes, the higher the health benefits. These plant foods purify and alkalize the body, while refined and processed foods can cause acidity and toxins to increase unhealthily.

But be aware that too much alkaline is also harmful. You need to know how to balance your diet with alkaline and acidic foods. After ingestion, hydrochloric acid in the stomach almost immediately neutralizes alkaline food and water. For your organ to work well, the balance between alkaline and acidic foods needs to be maintained.

A healthy and balanced diet is alkaline rather than acidic. Depending on your type of blood, the diet should consist of 60-80% alkaline foods and 20-40% acidic foods. Blood types A and AB normally require the highest level of the alkaline diet, while blood types O and B require more animal products in their diets. But remember, you're acidic when you're in pain.

The transition to an alkaline diet requires a change in one's food attitude. It is helpful to explore new tastes and textures and improve old habits.

Is there science behind the new fad diets?

Let us first look quickly at alkaline and acid to find out what the answer is and what it has to do with you?

All-natural foods contain acidic as well as alkaline elements. What are alkaline and acids? Acids are hydrogen-containing chemical compounds. Alkalinity is a measure of water's neutralizing capacity of acids. You are considered alkaline if you have pH values above seven. The pH measures a substance's acidity or alkalinity and stands for "potential hydrogen."

A pH of zero is fully acidic, and a pH of 14 is entirely alkaline. In short, we want your pH in your blood to be between 7.35 and 7.45 for your body to remain healthy. Outside this range, your body's activity is no longer optimal, and its metabolism is out of balance. Unfortunately, most people have and do not even realize high levels of acid.

The standard American diet does not include alkaline foods. Instead, they eat fatal animal products, grain, refined food, processed foods, carbohydrates, and sugars. When it is metabolized, inorganic and organic acids are produced and more than twice the amount of acid your bodies can handle.

These acids are all poisonous and must be removed as quickly as possible by your bodies. If the kidneys and large intestines eliminated these acids, the acid would damage your organ.

Most of your body's tissues are alkaline. Your body neutralizes natural mineral compounds to these acids. They neutralize each other when acid and alkaline are combined. The alkaline and the acid both disappear when this happens and water and a compound called salt appear in their place. Your bodies constantly go from acidic to alkalizing and back to the natural digestion process.

There is, however, a limit to this. If your blood is very acidic, oxygen and nutrients cannot be transported into your cells. To function properly, body cells need oxygen and nutrients. When we eat too many acidic foods or not enough foods, our cells may get sick and die.

Although your bodies hold alkaline reserves and are going to struggle to rebalance fluctuating levels without alkalization, the body draws the minerals from your bones and vital tissues from your alkaline mineral stores. Over time, mineral deficiencies in your bodies will cause serious health problems.

Stress, in addition to environmental toxins, GMOs, and drugs, can also make you acidic. How can you ensure that your body stays in a slightly alkalized state? To find the right balance, in addition to getting the right food, you need to evaluate your stress, trauma, and exercise habits.

Naturally grown and refined raw foods contain the nutrients and minerals necessary for a healthy, alkaline diet. Moreover, green supplements consisting of dried fruit and vegetables are popular to "alkalize the body."

Health Benefits

Today's food is completely different from our ancestors and is different from what we are used to today. How well we said, we are what we eat." The advance of technology has dragged us away with the kinds of food we consume.

A view of the grocery store shocks you with aisles of processed food and animal products. With the easy availability of fast foods today, finding one in our neighborhood is no difficult thing.

In recent years, animal products and refined food products have increased as the daily supply of fruits and vegetables is increasingly excluded from the diets. It is no surprise that many people are currently suffering from various kinds of illnesses and allergies, such as bone diseases, heart diseases, and many others. Some health professionals link these illnesses with the kind of food we eat.

Certain food types disturb the balance in our bodies that cause health problems in such cases. If we can only change our food habits, it is unlikely that disease prevention and health restoration can be achieved.

The alkaline and acid rations for a healthy body must be balanced and measured according to the body's pH level. The pH values are considered neutral between zero and 14 and seven. Any value below seven is considered to be acidic. Sophisticated foods, such as meat and meat derivatives, sweets, and some sweetened beverages, generate large amounts of acid on the body.

Acidosis is the common index of the different diseases that infect many people with high bloodstream and body cells' high acidic levels. Some health professionals conclude that acidosis is responsible for many people's critical diseases today.

An alkaline or alkaline diet usually neutralizes our body's high acid level to achieve a balanced state. This is the main function of the body's alkaline. The presence in the body of alkaline is quickly depleted because of the high acidic content to be neutralized, and alkaline food is insufficient to replenish the loss of alkaline

As previously described, acidosis causes many health problems. Critical acid level enters our system, breaking cells and organs if they do not correctly neutralize. To prevent this, a pH balance must be maintained.

It can be done with ease to test whether our body contains higher levels of alkaline. This is done with the use of pH strips from any pharmacy. Two types of strips exist, one for saliva and one for urine.

If you suffer from fatigue, headaches, and regular cold and flu, these symptoms indicate a high acid level in the body. Acidosis is how the body inhibits not only normal diseases, which we know, but high acid levels in the body cause other diseases that you may experience.

Depression, ulcers, high acidity, dry skin, acne, and overweight are some of the things connected to our body's extreme acidity. Other critical and severe diseases like osteoporosis, frequent infections, joint diseases, bronchitis, and heart disease are not limited.

Even with drugs, symptoms may be masked and continue to influence your health, as the root of the problem has not been eradicated. More medicines will only make the problem worse because the anti-inflammatory medicine will add to the body's acid level.

To attain the root of the diseases, our pH-value systems must be maintained in a healthy state. Alkaline foods that naturally occur in the body can supplement the lost alkaline in the neutralization process. By maintaining a healthy alkaline diet, the system replenishes enough alkaline, bringing the body to its predominant alkaline condition.

How then can an alkaline diet be incorporated into our eating habits?

The first very basic step is to reduce the intake of refined food. As we already know, these foods contain a large number of chemicals that increase our body acidity. The next step is to reduce the intake and amount of liquor of meat and its derivatives. The last step is to increase fresh fruit and vegetables because they are naturally high in alkalinity.

Oranges and lemons have become alkaline and absorbed by the body after digestion is a good alkaline diet. In general, we have to eat 75% of alkaline food daily. The more alkaline foods we put into our system, the greater the neutralization of our body's acidic condition.

CHAPTER 9

LIST OF ALKALINE FOODS - WHAT TO EAT FOR GOOD HEALTH

The pH range can be zero-14, and zero is the highest acidity and 14 the highest alkalinity. Our blood contains acid as well as alkaline residues in the food we eat. The ideal pH for a healthy person is, therefore, between 7.35 – 7.45. Even a slight decrease in this level can damage our cells, tissues, organs, and ultimately our system.

Our cells need nutrients and enzymes to survive, and the food we consume provides these essential nutrients. Some foods have higher acid levels, while other foods contain higher alkaline levels.

Acidic foods, naturally, will leave the residue of acid and are absorbed into our blood cells. Rather, alkaline-rich foods leave our cells with alkaline residues. There is a direct connection between proper consumption and maintaining a balanced pH.

Nature has given us an abundance of food. Fruits and vegetables are not limited to just a few sorts, so we don't have to be slow to eat the same thing every day. We don't have to take it by sticking to just one meal type to be fit and strong.

We need to determine the alkalinity and acidity levels of various foods and match them with our diets.

Anthony Robbins has a list of alkaline and acidic foods, so beginning this new diet approach should not be hard. We should understandably reduce our intake of acidic foods and beverages, especially if we have already reached the acidic limit.

Note that excessive acid levels in our system may cause serious diseases to develop. Yeah, we have to be mindful of what our bodies feed on. You will start making healthier food decisions not just for yourself but for your mates, using your list of alkaline foods.

To sustain a healthy pH is the underlying principle of the pH miracle diet. It is ideal for you to consume alkalizing foods because the human body is marginally alkaline. When you consume a little too much acidic foods, the digestive system becomes unbalanced. In turn, it causes many issues, including weight gain, depressed immunity, exhaustion, and low concentration, all of which can result in more severe health conditions.

Acidic foods (that are to be avoided), foods that are alkalizing (which are to be emphasized are the variables that affect the pH miracle diet. Alkalizing foods help maintain your body's pH and are, as a result, good for your body. Many people don't understand what pH, alkali, and acid mean and how they are associated with nutrition and health.

The properties of alkalinity and acidity are referred to as 'basic.' The cells that compose these foods decide these conditions. Therefore, the transition from alkaline to acid cannot be achieved by external treatment. Foods are alkaline or acidic at their foundation or base.

Chemically, alkaline and acidic compounds are opposites. If there is an interaction between an acid and a base, a salt occurs. In a chemist's laboratory, these interactions are clear and simple. However, the interaction is more complicated in our bodies due to the size with which the bases and acids meet.

In either case, scientists have made several generalizations about the effects of alkaline compounds and acids in our digestive system. In our body, acidic foods form acids. They reduce the pH of fluids, including saliva, lymph, and blood, and make them more acidic. Alkaline foods increase the pH number of these fluids and make them alkaline.

For general comparison, the 'standard' pH in human saliva is between 7.3 and 7.4. However, most people have less pH as they are more acidic. They are drained, burnt out, and their bodies starve for balance. Muscles are fatigued quickly under the influence of acidic foods. You are forced to slow down practically, as the body cannot produce the same results as before physically.

When you consume acidic foods, free radical degradation occurs, and this induces aging. Minerals and vitamins are not readily absorbed. The digestive system is thrown off balance as pleasant bacteria die.

Furthermore, the intestine's functions are impaired due to the acidity as nutrients are not absorbed so quickly. Cells become saturated with toxins that cannot be extracted. The majority of the systems in the body cannot work at maximum ability.

In comparison, alkaline foods are more beneficial to wellbeing. Eating such foods is more beneficial. They have antioxidant effects on the body. The assimilation at cellular levels is increased, and they enable the cells to function normally.

Yeast and parasitic growth are decreased due to these foods. Alkaline foods encourage more restful and deeper sleep, healthy and youthful skin, and help relieve suffering from colds, flu, and headaches. These foods also promote copious physical energy.

The link to cancer is a significant distinction between acidic and alkaline foods. Safe tissues are alkaline, while cancerous tissues are acidic. When oxygen combines with an acidic fluid, it forms water due to the combination with hydrogen ions. Though oxygen helps to neutralize the acid, the acid does not allow oxygen to reach the tissues.

The lone oxygen atom is open to move to another cell and extend the merits of oxygen to the other cells in the tissue. At a pH of over 7.4, cancer tissues become dormant. Studies have shown that, at pH 8.5, healthy tissues live while cancerous tissues die. There are many benefits to an alkalized diet, apart from preventing cancer.

To maintain good health, balanced body chemistry must also be used - this is highly necessary for maintaining a healthy lifestyle. Too much acidic foods cause what is known as 'acidosis.' They are a fundamental explanation for some diseases and particularly in persons with arthritic and rheumatic diseases that affect their joints.

You simply "burn" the food as you digest it - it becomes fuel just like a combustion engine turns gasoline into energy to propel you forward. Our fuel source is important in maintaining the balance of our health and our body, but if we have acidosis and an acidic diet, our body gets bad fuel.

You wouldn't bring diesel fuel into a normal vehicle, would you? You wouldn't, of course, because your body isn't any different.

We generate 'ash' as a by-product when our body burns fuel. This by-product may have several properties. They can be harmless, acidic, or alkaline - depending on the minerals in the food. This ash happens if the blood or tissue is poor in alkaline reserves.

We need to build a proportion of acid and alkaline to maintain a balance to keep our body in order. The average natural ratio is four parts of alkaline to one of acid or 80-20.

While we sustain these relationships, the body has extra strong disease tolerance and improved recovery, while when the balance is out of control, the opposite is true. Disease therapies should involve high alkaline foods so that acidity compensates them for the best chance of being beaten.

We have high alkaline reserves if our bodies are stable so that emergency needs can be easily met only if too much acid is swallowed. However, we will deplete these reserves, and our wellbeing can suffer significantly when the ratios start falling to three to one. We can operate normally, but only if we have enough alkaline in reserve and a correct alkaline ratio and acidic foods.

Five key alkaline foods help our bodies maintain the correct pH balance, and they are:

1. Broccoli - Broccoli is one of the vegetables we consume but not always know the great features that contribute to the circulation and fuel use.
2. Spinach – calorie spinach is by far, one of the best choices for alkaline foods with nutrients well beyond the norm.
3. Avocado - I love this fruit personally, and you know it is outstanding with reduced cholesterol and cardiovascular health.
4. Sprouts – Sprouts gives us several advantages, like cholesterol reduction and cardiac health help, but are also high in compounds that can strike cells that grow cancer.
5. Flaxseed Oil - This oil is rich in minerals that promote joint and bone health and can reduce arthritis in the short term by taking a tablet a day.

Eating plenty of alkaline foods every day will allow you to restore your body's pH balance to the best possible health.

CHAPTER 10
ALKALINE DIET FOR DIABETICS

In several respects, the human body is alkaline by nature. We allow it to work at an ideal level by keeping it alkaline. However, millions of metabolism reactions generate acidic waste as final products.

When we eat large quantities of acid-producing foods and inadequate alkaline food, we increase body acid toxicity. When we allow this acid waste to accumulate in the entire body, acidosis develops over time.

Acidosis will slowly weaken our body's essential functions if we do not take corrective measures quickly. Besides, acidosis is one of the leading causes of human aging. It leaves our body highly vulnerable to various lethal chronic diseases, including diabetes, cancer, arthritis, and heart diseases.

This is why the greatest challenge we humans face to protect our lives is to find the best way to minimize production and optimize body acid waste disposal. Our body needs a balanced lifestyle to prevent acidosis and age-related diseases and continue performing at the maximum possible rates.

This lifestyle will include daily workouts, a healthy diet, a clean physical environment, and a way of life that provides the lowest possible stress. A balanced lifestyle helps our body to preserve its acid waste content at the lowest possible level.

The alkaline diet appears to better suit the human body's nature. This is mostly because it helps to neutralize acid waste and to eliminate it from the body.

People should consider alkaline diets as general human dietary limits. Persons with special health conditions and medical needs will help adapt their needs to alkaline diet standards.

The miracle alkaline diet can help people with diabetes improve their overall health. Alkaline diets help improve body physiology and metabolism and their immune system, as they do with other humans.

This diet should help diabetics to regulate their blood sugar more effectively. It will also help decrease their weight gain and the risk of cardiovascular disorders and keep their cholesterol levels down.

Besides, the alkaline diet helps to better treat diabetes, making it easier for diabetics to prevent degenerative conditions. By adopting an alkaline diet, diabetics will at the same time live better and significantly increase their life expectancy, given their health conditions.

Generally speaking, people who choose to adopt an alkaline diet have to choose their daily foods on the Acid-Alkaline Food List.

A' Diabetics Acid-Alkaline Food Map' has been published recently. Using this particular graph, diabetics should comply with both the alkaline diet rule and the glycemic index rule.

The alkaline diet law sets general dietary guidelines. According to this diet plan, our daily food consumption must consist of at least 80% of the food derived from alkaline and not more than 20% of the acidifying foodstuffs.

Therefore, the more alkaline a food product is, the safer it is; on the other hand, the more acidifying a food product, the worse it will be for the human body.

As far as glycemic index laws are concerned, food is classified into four main groups regarding its capacity to raise blood sugar. The glycemic GI index ranges from zero to 100 now tests this ability.

1. Foods containing virtually no carbohydrates and which, as a result, have an insignificant glycemic index (GI~0).
2. Low glycemic carbohydrate foods (GI 55 or below); those with diabetes should consume these items with some caution.
3. Foods with high glycemic index carbohydrates (GI 56 or more); diabetics can, as far as possible, remove these from their diets.
4. Processed foods; diabetics may check the manufacturer's labels for their precise glycemic index values.

Further data are available on the Internet in the glycemic index of foods at the University of Sydney and the American Diabetes Association.

Diabetics Top Best and Top Worst Foods

The 'Diabetics Acid-Alkaline Food List' divides foods into six categories for those affected by diabetes. The following list ranges from the best to the worst foods.

1. Alkalizing GI~0 food products.

They are among the best ingredients. Diabetics will eat them free of charge.

Asparagus; broccoli; pets; celery; leftover; carob; vegetable juices; squash; okra; courgettes; cauliflower; garlic; green beans; beets; cod; raw spinach; lemons; avocados; lime; from chives; from herbal teas; stevia; from lemon water; from ginger tea; from green tea; toast oil; from olive oil; from flaxseed oil.

2. Dietary items with a GI of 55 or less.

Diabetes patients should be moderated, owing to their glycemic index.

Grass barley; sweet potato; carrots; new maize, olives; peas/soja; tomatoes; bananas, cherries; pears; orange peaches; mangoes; kiwi; papayas; berries; apples; mouthwash; Brazil's nut, rice; chestnuts; coconut; quinoa; hazelnuts; lentils; soy milk; soybeans; breast milk; raw honey; whey.

3. Acidifying GI~0 foods.

Diabetics should be careful to eat them because they are acid-producing.

Rhubarb; spinach cooked; pork; mollusks; liver; oysters; beef; poison; cold-water fish; chicken; turkey; eggs; butter; milk cottage; milk; maize oil; margarine; sunflower oil; wine; wine;

beer; coffee; tea; mayonnaise; mustard; vinegar; artificial sweeteners.

4. Foods with a GI of 55 or less are acidified.

Because of their acid-forming and glycemic levels, people with diabetes would have to eat them cautiously.

Lima beans; marine beans; kidney beans; pin tops; wheat-pastries; wheat; wheat; walnuts; squirrels; plums; brown rice; sprouted wheat-bread; maize; oat/rye; whole wheat/pastries; wheat; walnuts; peanuts; pistachios; carjacks; pecans; sunflower seeds; sesame; cream; yogurt; raw milk; custard; ice cream; homogenized Milk; chocolate.

5. Alkaline products with a GI of 56 or greater.

These goods are among the worst foods for diabetics due to their high glycemic index. Those with diabetes also ought to stop them.

Squid; beetroot; tofu; skin-like potato; fig; raw sugar; amaranth; millet; dates; melons; pineapple; watermelon; maple syrup; raw sugar.

6. Meat containing acid with a GI of 56 or higher.

Such products are too acidic and carbohydrate is too heavily glycemic. They are the worst food for diabetics. Diabetes sufferers also need to cut them off from their meals.

CHAPTER 11

HOW TO IMPROVE YOUR HEALTH EASILY WITH AN ALKALINE DIET

Many in the developed world have too acidic and overloaded toxins due to diet and stress factors. So, they face health issues that vary from mild or major skin irritations to depression, chronic fatigue, and back pain to arthritis, ulcers, osteoporosis, and cancer.

Just take the following facts into account:

Diseased bodies are unbalanced with high tissue and blood acidity concentration. Yet, our regular medical tests rarely detect the absence of this balance. Tests can show that you are all right, but otherwise, you feel.

Waste products left behind by inadequate digestion are the number one source of excess acidity. To digest our food, we need hydrochloric acid. The tougher a food is to digest, the more acid it needs to be digested.

In general, it is difficult to digest and means alkaline to form acids and easy to digest.

Well-being is easier to attain and sustain when you eat four times more alkaline foods than acidic foods. In maintaining such an optimal ratio, the body normally has healthy body chemistry and high disease tolerance.

SOLUTION: Find out what to eat to boost your wellbeing (and what to avoid)! The more alkaline food, with some exceptions, such as ulcer patients, allergy, and sugar sensitivity — who respond to sweet fruits or other particular foods are excellent for most.

Take a look at this list of alkaline and acidic foods to help you improve your health:

Higher foods become less alkaline and more acidic (usually more difficult to digest).

MORE ALKALINE: Best food, even good for detoxification.

A pinch of salt in the water of lemon/calamine

- Grassy Tea
- Honey (a little)
- Apple cider vinegar
- Coconut water
- Citrus fruit juice
- Further fruit juices
- Lactobacteria eat milk-free
- Farming fruits
- Sweet fruits
- Other fruits such as super mature bananas (except starchy fruits)

Green leafy fish and vegetables

All other crops (except two starchy veggies in the next category, and three listed at the bottom of the chart)

Flax, hemp, cocoon, and olive oil

SEMI-ALKALINE: Perfect for healthy citizens

- Tiny quantities of lactobacteria, goat's milk yogurt is best for dairy alone
- Blueberry
- Hot fruit and vegetables (potato, eggplant, normal banana, avocado, jackfruit, breadfruit)
- Ball screw nuts (in small quantity, blended or very well-chewed, not fried)
- Raw sugar

SEMI-ACID-FORMING: suitable in small amounts

- Sweetheart Theater (which is an herb, not a grain)
- Gently sprinkled vegetables (better use coconut oil) (better use coconut oil)
- Millet (the most alkaline grain) (the most alkaline grain)
- Other whole grain (including 100 percent bread/rice/noodles, maize, oats, and garlic)
- Tofu New
- Vegetables (e.g., lentils, mung beans, soy, peanut)

ACID-FORMING: For good people, a little is not that bad

Grains of refined consistency (including white rice, white bread white noodles, veggie-meat) (including white bread, white rice, white noodles, veggie-meat)

EXTREMELY ACID-FORM: Remove or minimize

- Profound fried foods
- Fish

- Poultry
- Meat

Eggs (hardest digestible food and bad cholesterol #1 source)

Notes:

1. Dairy goods vary from one's own – good for others, bad for others.
2. Refined sugar, tea, and coffee are not difficult to digest, but they form highly acidic and deprive the body of nutrients required to consume them in liberal terms.
3. Onion, garlic, and champagne are not difficult for absorption, but the lower drums heat up and sound rather unsettling.

Step up alkaline foods for your diet and see how your health improves!

CHAPTER 12

COMMON PLANT-BASED DIET MISCONCEPTIONS

Perhaps a vegetarian or vegan is the healthiest way to eat. However, people who consume meat in particular or sometimes mark vegetarians as low in frames or anemic or follow diets rapidly. However, some "myth-conceptions" are that people do not know how to eat a vegetable or vegan food. Many vegetables and fruits are high in protein and low in calories on the vegetarian menu.

Plant diets offer elite nutrition and health benefits, including lower risk of heart disease, carcinogenicity, and type 2 diabetes. In the Adventist Health Study 2, vegetables weigh 30 pounds less than meat-eaters on average. Eating veggies has great benefits, and it is important to learn the facts and reject myths.

The following myths and facts help you discover some "myth-conceptions" of a plant-based diet.

1: Fake Iron, Vegetarian and Vegan diets

Fact: The vegetarian or vegan diet comprises rich iron, such as dried apricots, mushrooms, dark green leafy food, beans, and fish.

2: Vegetarians are not getting a lot of protein

Fact: Many vegan foods contain enough protein, including beans and whole grains.

3: You can't adopt a vegetarian diet while you are pregnant.

Fact: The best way to provide your unborn baby with a vegetarian diet is to give pregnant women extra pounds after delivery. In addition to iron and calcium, bananas, legumes, cereals, and vegetables also supply fiber, which reduces bowel pain.

4: You can't follow a vegetarian diet if you're interested in sports.

Fact: Many athletes follow the successfully established vegetarian diet and receive the same amount of protein as high-food animal products from beans, wheat, and soy. Many athletes can eat almonds, walnuts, pistachio, grapes, cheese, eggs, sesame, pottery, black beans, lentils, and chickpeas quickly and easily. Quinoa is an excellent source of food and protein.

5: Kids are refusing to eat vegetarian or vegan

Fact: Some vegetarian foods include peanut butter, popcorn, and a wide variety of good fruit such as bananas, mule, kiwi, grapes, apples, oranges, and pears.

Fact: Tacos, cakes, and wraps are great, good vegan foods, and nutritious. Most kids will not reject this delicious, nutritious food.

6: Vegan or vegetarian foods are difficult to change

Fact: You don't radically move to a vegetarian or vegan way of life, but you may adjust to something in time. Make some changes and continue to enforce until animal products are eliminated.

You may try to make tacos instead of black beef, for example. You may omit chicken or stir-fry meat. You can fly comfortably via progressive innovations. There's a glass of warm champagne and a large dish: vegetable burgers, tofu sausage, you have bacon, all marvelous plates.

7: Vegetarians don't like animal products

Fact: Vegetarians don't always consume safer meat. They don't complain about the use of animal by-products like leather or fur. On the other hand, vegetables typically have abandoned derivatives of meat and livestock. The use of animal products such as honey and hair, silk, and leather is usually not encouraged. Veganism is not a way of life or an ideology.

8: Vegetarian and vegan diets should also be considered

Fact: B-12, available only for red meat, fish, milk, and eggs, is the only supplement required for vegan feeding. The important vitamins of vegetarians and vegetables are obtained by grain, vegetables, plants, and fruits (B-grouping, A, E, C). Many vegetarian and vegan diets are also rich in iron and calcium.

9: Vegetarians are not getting enough protein.

Fact: Most Americans eat too much protein. This can have severe health consequences that can lead to kidney disease, osteoporosis, and cardiac disease.

10: Vegetarians are skinny, weak, about 98 pounds.

Fact: Isn't it interesting how some of the biggest mammals on Earth are plant food eaters like gorillas and cows? When people eat dead animals, the protein and other nutrients are taken secondhand. The cow or the pig has eaten plants, which are the real powerhouses of nutrients.

11: Vegetarians eat potatoes.

Fact: Some people seem to be advancing or stuck in a certain stage during the evolution of their dietary habits. They think chicken doesn't count as meat for some reason. Or they don't think white meat" counts. Chicken and beef contain similar cholesterol amounts.

12: Vegetarians are not getting enough calcium.

Fact: They do not have to eat as much calcium by eliminating animal products from their diets. High acid foods such as meat pull calcium out of the bones to return blood to homeostasis with the correct calcium balance. A negative calcium balance, not the lack of milk in the diet, contributes to osteoporosis. Calcium-fortified soy milk and juice, calcium-set tofu, soybean and soy, broccoli, collards, Chinese cobblestone, kale, mustard greens, and okra are good plants for easily absorbed calcium.

13: Vegetarians cannot eat out.

Fact: Years ago, people who did not eat meat could have had difficulty eating in restaurants. But that's just no longer true. More and more restaurants are including light and vegetarian menus. Some fast-food restaurants, including Burger King, have a veggie burger.

14: Vegetarians eat fish.

Fact: Like number three, it seems that people don't think that fish is a species. These people are known as fishmongers. For omega-3 fatty acids, fish is sometimes eaten. Flaxseed, however, offers a better option. The oceans are overfished, and toxins like mercury often infect fish. It is high in cholesterol, too.

15: Vegetarianism is a fad of a new age.

Fact: Like artists, new-age people often see light before society's rest. Some vegetarians are great junk food eaters, but many have changed their diets to one based on plants and are healthier than the population.

When they turn to an herbal diet, many people are fascinated by all the new food options before them and consume more variety. This helps to improve their health and vitality.

16: Vegetarians are deluded into living forever.

Fact: You might not live longer if you are a vegetarian. But you would most definitely feel good when you are alive rather than wasting your time and money in the doctor's office.

CHAPTER 13

THE BEST FOODS AND SUPPLEMENTS FOR STARTING YOUR DETOXIFICATION JOURNEY

Today, people are aware that they should be hale and hearty; to clean up their bodies, they use raw foods to be detoxified. Since they give antioxidants, vitamins, nutrients, and detoxification, which are lost during the cooking process, it is better to quickly gain detoxification from high heat.

Most diseases are caused by the presence of too many toxins in the body. To have a healthy body, the body's toxins must be removed. In the following passage, you will be exposed to three types of food with a detoxification effect.

The liver's main function is to decompose and remove all the metabolic waste products and the chemical toxins we eat and drink utilizing our food. Phase I and phase II are the two detoxification routes, and the diet we use helps to control and complement the detoxifying activities.

When these toxins are stocked up in the body and are not removed immediately, they cause different kinds of health problems to the immune system, glandular system, and nervous system. This makes it all the more important to eat food that facilitates smooth liver detoxification. Here are the top five foods for detoxification.

Food is ideal for well-being, but the mystery remains that it is the best for cleansing and detoxification. We have a proper system for cleaning and detoxifying our bodies to eliminate toxins in the bloodstream.

This often results in an inconvenience that can be felt in many ways. Symptoms of flu and dull muscles are noticeable - yes, a healing crisis. Nevertheless, we must clean to alleviate tension.

Below are raw foods that have been declared most successful for detoxification and have been proven to help people boost their overall health, increase their resilience, lose weight, and increase their survival chances.

1. **Broccoli**, a cruciferous vegetable, has glucoraphanin as its phytonutrient, improving the lumber detox enzymes to clear substances known to cause cancer.

2. **Cilantro** – also called coriander, will purify your body from harmful bacteria such as salmonella and reduce mercury levels effectively.

3. **Prunes** - Prunes are a renowned source of soluble fiber and other nutrients and are beneficial in chronic constipation treatment and overall digestive system health improvement.

4. **Garlic** - Aged garlic, in particular, can accelerate the liver enzymes to filter out the digestive system's toxic deposits.

5. **Onions** - Like garlic, this allium vegetable is a strong detoxifying agent that encourages the liver to generate more enzymes when the digestive tract is eliminated due to bacterial infestations.

6. **Green Tea** - An ancient remedy in China and many Asian countries, green teas are known for preventing skin-aging free radicals. These antioxidants are your defense against free radicals and chemicals that can hurt you and make you look aged. Green tea also contains another form of antioxidants called catechins that have been shown to increase the liver's function.

7. **Seeds** - Fiber in flaxseeds, pumpkin seeds, hemp seeds, sesame seeds, chia seeds, and sunflower seeds help reduce harmful contaminants in the body. Furthermore, these seeds contain Omega-3 EFA suitable for reconstructing damaged tissues caused by free radicals.

8. **Nuts** - usually the best sources of the antioxidant, immune, and nerve protective vitamin E. Nuts are rich sources of essential fatty acids, healthy fats that minimize blood pressure. Besides, nuts have many more nutrients than tone and improve body resistance to disease.

9. **Omega-3 Oils** - Ideally, consume crude avocado, virgin olive oils, or flax oil during detoxification. This helps to lubricate the intestinal walls and to absorb toxins from the oil and remove them in the body.

10. **Artichoke** - Just one of the best detox foods, artichokes increase liver bile content. It also helps to cleanse and defend the liver against possible bacterial

or viral threats. Likewise, artichokes damage the kidneys diuretically.

Cynarine, a compound especially concentrated in the leaves, is the responsible component in artichokes. Cynarine is found to decrease cholesterol along with another compound, luteolin. Artichoke extracts treat irritable bowel syndrome and other gastrointestinal disorders effectively.

Eat Cilantro, Drink Lime

Continue to drink freshly squeezed lime juice for hydration during the day. What heals you most is a fruit breakfast with plenty of vitamins and minerals. These fibers are like brushes that purify the colon and intestines of your area.

If you want the strength to fly, just try cilantro, one of the most effective detoxifiers. So during your lunch, make it a habit for cilantro to be blended into a drink to help extract toxins from your body. You should apply it to a salad with a gingery dressing . Ginger is anti-inflammatory and allows gastric juices to help you digest.

Go on a diet for salad

During your salad diet, eat cabbage, beetroot, courgette, red pepper, white chops, and spring onions. Use new mint dressing and coriander to feel refreshing. To help you detoxify, include foods rich in vitamins E B6and C, potassium, nitrates, folate, beta-carotene, and fiber. So next time you get these unhealthy food cravings, immerse yourself in nutritional alternatives for a filling experience.

Why go organic?

Combine them during meals with juices and herbal teas. It is even better if the food is organic - processed by natural cultivation methods and free from harmful chemicals such as synthetic fertilizers and pesticides.

Now, what is the best detoxifying food if we take the organic path? Take sulfur-rich garlic, for instance, to help the body release all toxic compounds. It improves the liver's role in developing these enzymes, which remove toxins from the bloodstream.

Fruits and greens to cleanse

Apple is a source of minerals, fibers, vitamins, and phytonutrients. It makes bile production in the liver easier to detoxify. They have soluble pectin fibers that bind to the blood and intestines, heavy metals, and cholesterol.

Leafy greens, such as broccoli, chocolate, kale, and spinach, are antioxidants that eliminate harmful byproducts from one's body. Avocado is excellent for the elimination of carcinogens from our bodies.

You know that detoxification happens when the blood becomes smaller than the lymphatic fluid.

Grapefruit – Grapefruit is rich in two good liver cleansers, natural vitamin C, and antioxidants. It also contains naringenin that helps the liver to burn and not store fat.

Garlic - Garlic contains high levels of compounds, including allicin and selenium that contribute to liver cleansing and protect the liver against toxicity damage.

Green Tea - Green Tea is filled with catechins, a potent antioxidant found in studies to minimize liver fat accumulation and promote proper liver function.

Lemon & Lime - These two citrus fruits have very high vitamin C levels that help the body turn toxic materials into water-absorbed substances. Drinking morning freshly squeezed lemon or lime juice often improves the role of the bowel and liver.

Avocado – This nutrient-dense superfood allows the body to grow glutathione, promoting liver health, and improving its cleaning ability by shielding it from toxic overload.

Walnuts - Walnuts contain high levels of l-arginine, glutathione, and omega-3 fatty acid, which help detoxify the liver and cause it. They also assist in blood oxygenation.

Turmeric - Turmeric has been shown to effectively protect the liver against toxic damage and regenerate damaged liver cells, one of the most productive foods to maintain a healthy liver. Turmeric also stimulates natural bile development, shrinks hepatic ducts, and improves the gallbladder's overall function, another organ that purifies the body.

Leafy Greens – Our most popular liver cleaning partners can be eaten raw, fried, or juiced with the leafy greens. Quite abundant in plant chlorophylls and phytonutrients, greens suck up blood pollutants. These cleaning foods have a good protective mechanism for the liver through their distinct ability to neutralize heavy metals, toxins, and pesticides.

Apples - Pectin-rich apples contain the chemical components necessary to clean up and release toxins from the digestive tract. In return, this enables the treatment of toxic load by the liver during the washing process.

Broccoli & Cauliflower - The cruciferous plants increase the amount of glucosinolate in the system, contributing to enzyme liver production. These enzymes help minimize cancer risk by removing carcinogenic compounds and other toxins in the body.

Almonds are good for stabilizing blood sugar. They are good fiber, calcium, and natural protein sources.

Apples are also used to detoxify the body. It helps to cleanse the intestines. Apples are also strongly anti-inflammatory, anti-bacterial, and anti-cancerous. These benefits include reducing cholesterol levels and preventing cancer. Pectin helps the body excrete dietary toxins, including synthetic asthma-related chemicals and hyperactivity in young children.

Bananas are also used for body purification. It helps to calm and reinforce the abdomen. Bananas are rich in minerals essential to optimal washing. Potassium helps to control the fluid in the body and reduce the build-up of tissue fluid. It also has many antibacterial properties that lead to the elimination of harmful bacteria in the intestine.

Avocados play various important functions, such as reducing cholesterol, vessel dilation, and destruction of toxicity. Compounds are used in avocados to treat 30 types of carcinogenic substances. Avocados also benefit the liver and are used to prevent arthritis, a disease.

Blueberries have rich antibacterial and anti-viral properties that prevent the effects on the tissue of chronic inflammation, which at the same time minimize pain.

Artichokes support bile growth. Bile helps the bowels to destroy toxins in the body.

Celery and spinach are perfectly used to detox the body, while celery helps lower hypertension. It is also rich in anti-cancer properties that help to drive cancer cells out of the body.

Kelp includes a substance called "polysaccharide sulfate" capable of removing cholesterol attachment from the vessel's wall to maintain natural cholesterol levels. Kelp alginate can form a gelatin layer in the intestines that can prevent the body from consuming harmful contaminants such as plum, cadmium, and other heavy metals and remove radioactive materials from the body.

It is also effective in atherosclerosis treatment and can prevent constipation and colon cancer. Kelp also contains a lot of iodine, which can stimulate hypophysis, thereby reducing the hormone levels in women, restoring the ovaries, and removing the hidden hazards from breast hyperplasia.

Carrot is a major detox in food. When combined with body mercury ions, the body will decrease mercury ions and increase these mercury ions. Carrots can help prevent hardening of the artery and lower body cholesterol levels.

Carotene in carrots can remove free radicals that can help people age. It also provides some other nutrients, such as vitamins B and C, which are also anti-aging. Carrots can also decrease the prevalence of ovarian cancer in women.

Traditional medicine also suggests that as fungal products grow in a cool and humid atmosphere, they are affected by nutritional vitality and blood circulation and can minimize toxic heat in the blood.

The plant pectin in the black fungus can absorb waste and contaminants from the human digestive system to purify the intestines and stomach. The black fungus can support the digestion of food and is highly successful in treating kidney and gallstones. Furthermore, black fungi can suppress blood clots and prevent thrombosis.

1. Fresh vegetables and berries: Fresh fruit and vegetables help both phases I and phase II detox methods. They are rich in antioxidants, which help to protect the liver against damage caused by toxic substances. It has been found that organic vegetables are more effective.

2. Important fatty acids: The body would have to consume fresh seeds and nuts, and they're unheated and cold-pressed oils. The use of hydrogenated fats in many processed foods must be avoided.

3. Sulfur: The sulfur content of foods, including eggs, beef, garlic, onion, radish, and turnips, is very important and is very useful in the phase II detox path.

4. Cruciferous vegetables: These vegetables help the liver turn various carcinogenic chemicals into less toxic compounds washed from the body. In the phase II detoxifying method, chicken, cool, broccoli, radish, turnip, and many others are helpful.

5. Good quality protein: egg, fish, and meat give the body enough amino acids required for the phase II detox.

Only healthy foods should be consumed so that the body is not further burdened with harmful substances.

If you care about your eating habits and help the liver with the right foods, your consumption will better and function efficiently.

Alcohols directly poison our bodies and saturate them with toxic toxins and other malnutrition, among other beverages and foods.

For example, processed foods are usually packed with saturated fat, salt, sugar, and artificial flavors, colors, and preservatives, making them as nourishing as a piece of carton. It is true, and it is probably better to eat a piece of cardboard than to eat much of the packaged snack foods out there. The following foods can:

- Make us experience weight gain
- Can cause us to be sick
- Make us feel bad and lack energy

These foods can also raise our risk of heart disease and diabetes. As a result, many people try to eliminate toxic toxins from their bodies and adopt some kind of detox diet to help them lose weight and feel healthier in the process.

These are some of the most useful foods, beverages, and supplements that detoxify the body.

Water - Water is important to our body's safe work. We can go without food for weeks as humans, but we will be fortunate to live without water for more than 48 hours. For us, this is how critical it is.

The human body consists of almost 80% water and is essential for our vital organs. To rid our species of toxic chemicals, we must drink plenty of water . The indication is in the word "flush" the body's toxins. A lot of water needs to be ingested to complete a successful detox.

Olive Oil - The saturated fat and essential fatty acids are high in olive oil. These fatty acids make our bodies incredibly balanced. It also has a host of other healthy properties, including strong antioxidants and minerals.

All the vitamins, minerals, and antioxidants are safe and allow our bodies to function fully, and our immune system to the maximum. Our immune system helps us prevent illness, disease, and infection.

Broccoli is another food filled with vitamins and minerals. It is considered a "super-food," and it's no wonder that it's one of the most powerful anti-cancer foods to hope for. Broccoli contains enzymes that allow your liver to transform harmful toxins into something that your body can flush toxins out of your system incredibly quickly. Make sure it doesn't microwave because radiation will kill some of the natural goodness it contains.

Meal replacement and weight loss supplements - You need something that includes a bit of everything that you need if your body is to detoxify and get rid of harmful toxins fully.

Yeah, the foods we've mentioned above help detox your body, but what about incorporating all of its detoxifying properties and much more to produce a meal replacement supplement that detoxifies your body and delivers a heap of vitamins, minerals, and antioxidants, and helps you lose weight?

The best detox diets are designed to be healthy and incorporate natural nutrients to the loss of weight. They should be full of good natural ingredients. Follow these steps, and it will be quick, efficient, and above all, easy to follow the best detox diets.

75

CHAPTER 14

DETOXIFICATION - WE ARE NOT EATING THE RIGHT FOODS FOR OUR BODY TYPE

Centuries ago, we used to kill for food, but today meat is being processed and has lost much of its nutritional value. People used to eat fruit and berries before picking them, so we go to the grocery store to buy our fruit and vegetables.

As soon as vegetables and fruits are picked, they are not delivered to the grocery store for longer than we know. The grocery stores were in bulk cheers and kept the fruits and vegetables at warehouses until it is shipped to the store, if possible. Weather influences fruit and vegetable prices too, so much that we don't consume as much fruit and vegetable as we can because of a lack of abundance of volatility.

Today, schools serve students breakfast and lunch. While they have some dietary standards to comply with, they also provide students with packaged, unhealthy food, which also causes unhealthy eating habits.

Since schools serve so many pupils both at breakfast and at lunch, they still need to obey those rules; our children have learned to have poor eating habits and then continue to eat poorly. This is why in adulthood and beyond, we still see more health issues.

The creation of good eating practices begins when parents prepare nutritional meals and teach children how to balance fruits, vegetables, meats, chicken, fish, and bread for nutritional meals and build a healthy menu throughout the month.

You must also suggest listening to your body when it tells you what it needs to support itself. For example, some people should have more fish and chicken in their diet and the amount of fluid we take every day.

We must also learn how various foods influence our bodies. For example, your body can not tolerate many acidic food types. If you do not have any certain vitamin deficiency in your body and eat high-acid fluids like pineapple juice or orange juice, it can also adversely affect you, with sores on the face.

You must also note that some things you consume can have parasites that can cause health issues like allergies, stomach problems, or chronic diseases such as fibromyalgia or bowel syndrome. In this scenario, you need to think about how you can detoxify products if you use these toxins in your body.

Many people who grow up in various cultures consume food abundant in that culture, and then they prefer to eat the same food habits with them when they migrate to different countries. A broad chain of grocery stores tend to transport food based on the people who live in the city.

As grocery stores use computerized scanners at checkout counters, they can calculate which goods are sold in various stores to a higher volume and determine what they bought for transport in those stores.

When you grow up to eat nutritious food and exercise regularly, it becomes part of your everyday routine, reducing obesity and increasing your life expectancy. Our forefathers ate more healthily than we do today, but only because they lived at an early age; they lived shorter lifetimes.

Even if we are advanced today because we rely on food raised on the farm, but because more people feed it, we have been able to process food in greater quantities, which has produced unhealthy eating habits and has also caused obesity and more health challenges. In our society, we must learn how to combat these evil habits, or we will see the life expectancy of all our children diminish.

Detoxification helps to eliminate contaminants from the body and rejuvenate your overall health. You need to undergo a detox program to prevent complications such as colon cancer, constipation, diabetes, bloating, etc., at least once a month.

There are various ways to naturally detoxify the body, such as juice cleanses, enema, etc. These processes help greatly cleanse your colon and thus nourish your digestive tract. The washing of columns not only helps to prevent sickness but also facilitates loss of weight.

It can easily throw away the stubborn abdominal fats. Before these detox treatments, it is often advised to consult a doctor. You should also have a balanced lifestyle to achieve better results. You should drink at least 10-12 glasses of water a day to keep the body hydrated and free of toxins.

Complete Body Detox Foods

* Foods containing fibers are the best way to safely and naturally detoxify the body. The best bet for colon cleaning is green leafy vegetables. It is highly recommended that you eat them raw for maximum advantages. You can add it to the juices too.

* The citrus fruits contain vitamin C, which can easily convert contaminants into water-soluble. The ultimate natural detox food is the fresh lemonade.

* You can also add garlic to set off liver enzymes that can discard panache garbage.

* To flush out the toxins in your body, you can use green tea. Catechins and antioxidants are abundant.

* Psyllium is rich in fiber which can mix up cholesterol and toxins easily.

* Various foods can be consumed naturally for detoxification, such as broccoli, sesame seeds, watercress, etc.

CHAPTER 15

BREAKDOWNS OF THE BODY'S NATURAL DETOX PROCESS

The air we breathe in is profoundly influenced by the atmosphere in which we live. If there is a factory near the place where you mostly live, you will possibly get toxins dispersed during the manufacturing process.

These factors taint the water we drink in one way or another. Although with safety labels and considered healthy and safe, the food that we eat can also contain toxins that are harmful in one way to our bodies.

Our body has a good way to detoxify itself. These toxins are expelled from our bodies by various organs, such as the skin by sweating, the kidney by urination, and the liver, which transforms and dumps different toxins.

Even if our body can detoxify itself without assistance, the pure amount of toxins we get every day can often overpower our natural detoxification regime. How do we help our body eliminate these dangerous toxins without costing us a leg and an arm?

Without understanding it, we allow our body to detox faster than normal. Drinking plenty of water would preferably help us urinate more often by drinking eight glasses a day or more. A sauna workout or trip will allow us to transpire more.

A health-conscious individual who consumes and claims that fruits and vegetables are already helping themselves detox naturally by not adding harmful toxins into the body from unhealthy foods. Ask anyone you know who never eats pork if they even have a tiny slice of it.

You will respond that your body particularly feels sick, your stomachs bad, and you will feel itchiness on your skin. This is because pork meat itself is fat and contains many contaminants because of how pigs are cultivated and the climate in which they live.

These same health-conscious people also contribute to toxic toxins' detoxification as certain vegetables and fruits fall under fibrous foods. Fibrous foods significantly contribute to our metabolism and bowel movement. If an individual is constipated frequently, it might circulate back into one system instead of flushing the toxins out during bowel movement.

Although these toxins can be good for our system, we should not overdo it because a disorder called the Herxheimer reaction is ultimately too rapid to remove the toxins compared with how our body disposes of them naturally. Symptoms include headaches, nausea, contraction of the bowel, and vomiting. Only mildly detox your body to keep one step ahead of every day's ever-growing toxins.

Knowing when natural detoxification should start

Body aches, daily tiredness, and intestinal stress indicate the need for natural detoxification of the body. You may have heard about detox services. If you suffer from any symptoms above, you may have wondered if it might benefit you. Here are questions to ask before you start a detox program:

- Do I ever feel tired, even though I'm not physically stressed?
- Do I drink six to eight glasses of water a day?
- Do I have sleep problems because of low backaches or cramps?

Answering yes to these questions suggests that detoxification of the body will be helpful.

A short description of natural methods of detoxification

Many people who choose to detox prefer to do this with a special diet. Others fill up on a juice or liquid easily. Some complete a colonic, where waste is disposed of by gentle irrigation. You should select the approach that best suits your needs and level of comfort.

Preparation for the method of natural detoxification

You are ready to embark on a wonderful process that will cleanse your body and detoxify your liver. You can prepare your body and mind for detox by performing many simple acts.

- Keep a newsletter.
- Drink water in abundance.
- Swimming, Walking, biking, or going to the gym.
- Speak to your family and friends about what you can do.
- Write down all your thoughts about detox and speak to a friend about it

You would want to try foods with a high content of fiber. It is natural and healthy and can help you to get healthier. See more now. Find more today.

Excellent ways to expand the natural detoxification benefits

A detox diet can improve your overall health dramatically and boost your mood. You will continue to reap the benefits while your detox diet finishes. Continue to eat carefully and keep your food log up to date.

Writing your food intake reflections will help you to break down bad habits. Complete your everyday routine with plenty of fresh fruit and vegetables. They make excellent dinner services, breakfast, and snacks. Remember to show compassion as you loop in new good habits. Dwell on the good ones, not the poor ones. We are all growing up despite our mistakes.

The FDA has not assessed these claims. These products should not be used for diagnosing, treating, curing, or preventing any disease.

Do I still have to detox the body, this is a question posed by a lot of people who are highly aware of their health. Thanks to the burden put on people, many people will detoxify their bodies to eliminate the extra fat. However, detoxification is not just a means of losing weight; you can naturally kill toxins through a completely effective natural detoxification method.

Most people don't care about what they eat and drink. Indeed the misuse of nicotine and alcohol, which their bodies and the chemicals already in the environment cause, already contributes to various health problems. Besides, you may have a caffeine addiction. Depression and anxiety are also reasons that so many people have an accumulation of toxins in their bodies.

This means they don't eat and drink well. If you suffer from this problem and feel depressed and lethargic, you may want your body's full detoxification. The best approach is to find short-term methods of detoxification.

Did you find that your digestive system doesn't function at the highest efficiency to keep you healthy?

Your immune mechanism is yet another system that is impaired by the accumulation of toxins. Your metabolism also generates a significant number of toxins, such as your kidney, liver, gallbladder, and digestive systems, in the bio-physiology of your organ and functions.

Both the kidney and liver are instrumental in the frequent and systematic elimination of any extra waste.

So how do you detox your body absolutely, you may ask?

Cut down the intake of caffeine, alcohol, and tobacco first. Your job is to rid yourself of all accumulated contaminants, including alcohol and nicotine. A successful detoxification method consists of organically grown fruit, and vegetables consumed raw or made into fresh juice.

Make sure that no residual toxins are added to your diet. There will only be a healthy detox diet for around three to four days. It's about time the body needs to get rid of toxins and dead tissue.

Today, there are a large number of detoxification services on the market. It is, therefore, only normal to be uncertain about which detoxification program is most suitable for your body. There are also various body cleaning diets, and I want to tell you about some of them to get the basic idea.

First and foremost, when using a detoxification program, you can fully eliminate the use of sugar, caffeine, refined foods, and alcohol. This effectively helps the body eliminate the accumulated toxins. It should be remembered that any diet changes should be promptly informed of a doctor; only if the doctor approves it will it continue.

Having juices in your everyday diet is also one of the easiest ways to detox your body naturally. A variety of juice diets and beverages are known to detoxify the body effectively. However, not all diets you make are beneficial for your body.

There are vehemently alternative drugs on the market that also help clean the body. Such drugs can enable the body to extract the garbage over time. These drugs have discussed energy problems, taking care of the mind and body while detoxifying them.

Practices such as acupuncture, acupressure, and Qi Gong are also useful in treating detoxification issues. It takes time to detoxify your body completely, and thus, patience is the secret to using a detoxification program for your body.

It is a fact that the most successful and common ideas of detoxification come from the use of water. As you know, three-fourths of our body is composed of water, so it is clear that drinking plenty of water naturally fills the body's contaminants with urine and transpiration. This is why doctors prescribe eight glasses of water per day to detoxify the body.

Water also preserves the body's normal balance and removes the body's toxins. Furthermore, no detoxification regimen is entirely effective if you do not drink optimal water with it. The explanation is that it is very difficult for our body to remove all the harmful compounds in the right water level, which does not keep the body sluggish and slow.

Natural products and methods must always be selected to speed up the body's cleansing process, not wait for the body to complete its detoxification. Full body detox is the most accurate way to avoid infections and diseases. A complete body clearing includes various bowel, liver, digestive, lymphatic, lung, and skin sections.

For this purpose, services covering these bodies must be chosen. Detox services typically require a change in dietary patterns. This means that a person needs to improve nutrition and prevent and eliminate toxins. He needs to strengthen the digestive system by utilizing balanced diets.

If you want to detox your body naturally, then a full body detox must be maintained daily. It helps the system neutralize and remove all toxins stored in various species with permanent total detoxification. Sustainable body washing certainly helps to clear the colon and hold the body in a continuous detox.

If this detox process is not conducted frequently, the body will likely retake new contaminants that become dysfunctional health. Furthermore, it can induce some medical problems such as a low immune system when the body increases toxins. It is important to choose methods for certain detoxifying sections of the body.

The ingestion of raw, steamed, or partially fried food, such as vegetables, fruit, sprouted seeds, soups, jus, and cereals, is part of any natural detoxification process. Continuous detoxification aims to encourage good health and avoid potential diseases. The majority of natural approaches include special diets, medications, and natural supplements such as herbal products.

Mediterranean diets are effective since they are low in carbohydrates and fat incorporated into a complete diet. Choosing organic diets, daily exercises, and enough fluids to speed up the detox process is also helpful.

Exercise is among the best ways to detoxify your organs. In general, this process combines oxygen therapy with hyperthermia that encourages body detoxification if a person sweats during the daily workout. To maximize its efficacy, exercise is prescribed three days a week so that organs such as the lungs, heart, and bowels can be assisted to remove harmful toxins.

There are many fitness programs and plans for people of all lifestyles and ages available in this regard. One good way to start is to walk 12 or 15 minutes a day to strengthen the colon.

However, it is often easier for our bodies to spontaneously detoxify if we have good eating habits, daily exercise, ample water, and a suitable lifestyle. This way, our mind, and body will remain completely safe and balanced.

Now that you know the advantages of full-body detoxification, you want a detoxification plan that involves a natural diet and other diets that help detoxify your body. These detox remedies must be taken at least once a year to clear up all the accumulated waste from your body.

CHAPTER 16

THE MAIN BENEFITS OF NATURAL DETOXIFICATION

The natural detoxification process is where the body of harmful toxins and unnatural additives are purified naturally. These are toxins and substances we come in contact with or eat because of our western lifestyle. This means a serious change to our food and drink in our bodies. These foods or drinks usually have more than a nutrition advantage but are natural eliminators.

The lungs, intestinal tract, urinary system, skin, and lymph system perform the body's natural detoxification every day. This would be enough for the body's requirements for normal purposes and in a clean and sober world.

In all this, water is also a necessary tool. We don't drink enough pure water in our modern world, and some people never drink plain water! The result is severe dehydration for most people.

Naturally, organic fruits and vegetables should be consumed as a raw food diet and drinking more water. There should be no animal products (including milk and eggs) and as little refined and cooked food (especially fried) as possible.

There should be exercise, not extreme, but regular low-level aerobic exercise during the detoxification process, which will make you sweat. This also improves bowel movements considerably.

Following the above simple methods, the whole body is cleaned naturally, including colon detox, and helps in the natural detoxification of alcohol and drugs, including marijuana. Some people will fast naturally for these purposes, but this is not needed if you follow a detailed plan over a certain period with certain rules and advice on what you should not eat.

The dilemma is what curriculum to follow or plan to follow. It is pointless to purchase and expect a natural detoxification diet plan with herbal pills. Some decent detox plans are available online, but some aren't so good, so you have to go to a comparison site that lists the best. Read on to find this below.

Toxin exposure in this modern-day lifestyle is inevitable

Health is rich, or at least this is what some people claim, but it can be a challenge to maintain an effective immune system, especially when considering toxins that invade our everyday life. Thousands of chemical compounds and toxins enter our homes and places of work.

The food we eat, the water we drink, the air we breathe are free radicals. The traditional daily diet consists of refined food, sugar, and fats that affect the immune system's efficacy. The invasion of free radicals leads to health problems.

The body has a natural detox mechanism. The liver, kidneys, and bowels continually filter and extract the nasty contaminants that alter the cells and molecules in any body organ.

Although the liver is healthy, it cleanses the body and prevents contaminants from entering the bloodstream; it weakens the immune system when the internal organs are filled with toxins.

The natural detox mechanism slows down as free radicals are bound to cells in the body. Toxins are present in fat cells made up all over the body and in the brain, liver, and colon cells. The cells are modified, and the body is vulnerable to some health problems.

Start the natural process of detoxification of the body

Detox also describes the removal of alcohol or narcotics from a recovery center. Still, free radicals may also be detoxified from the internal system through diet change, colon cleansing kits, master cleansing juice, and herbal cleansing.

One healthy way to clean up the colon is to quickly consume fresh fruits and vegetables, drink plenty of water, and add herbal tea to your diet for a few days. Eliminate foods from the process to prevent alcohol, tobacco, sugar, and reduce the amount of caffeine you eat.

There is colon cleanses that clean the colon quickly on the market in relatively short a week or ten days, but those bought cleaning kits may not be successful in the long term unless a change in the daily diet occurs.

The first step in the natural detoxification process is the healthy detoxification of all internal organs. A safe cleanse requires at least 435 minutes per week of exercises and hydrotherapy to improve blood flow and dry-skin brushes to strengthen the skin. The skin is another essential organ to purify, especially if you want a clear hue.

Cleaning quickly means successful cleaning and detoxification through a body detoxification program that involves essential vitamins, fruits and vegetables, plenty of water and juice, and some kind of exercise in the body and mind. Health is wealth when you naturally detox the body.

Detoxification is a mechanism by which to purify the body of toxins and harmful chemicals. It includes dietary and behavioral changes that reduce and increase the intake of toxins. These toxins are primarily caused by food, medicine, and exposure to the environment and are difficult to eliminate. In this method, natural detoxification is beneficial.

Mother Nature's natural detoxification method typically suffices for good health. This system protects us against regular toxin exposure. The respiratory (bronchial tube, lungs, sinus, and nose), gastrointestinal (gall bladder, liver, colon), urinary (kidneyurethra, bladder), dermal (sebaceous glands sweat, and tears), and lymph system (lymph nodes and canals), are part of the human detoxification system.

The human body is designed to tackle toxic attacks at low levels. Our bodies can detoxify possible carcinogenic compounds or repair genetic damage. The protective mechanisms include repair, cell removal, detox, and nutritional antioxidants. The human body can detoxify if it is fed properly with fiber and water.

Water is our body's primary detoxifying agent. It helps us cleanse our skin and kidneys and increases sweating by exercising. Many of us are chronically dehydrated, and physicians prescribe at least eight water glasses a day.

The next step is a raw-food diet of natural detoxification. This means more fruit and vegetables and less protein and fat-rich red meat, milk, processed food, and fried food. Adding fiber to your diet helps to detoxify your system periodically.

Regular exercise is another essential component of natural detoxification. Exercise alleviates sweating contaminants from the body and also aids in healthy bowel behavior. Exercise increases our overall metabolism and helps detoxify. Aerobic activity helps hold the body sound.

Some natural therapists also recommend treating the gastrointestinal system with waste and hazardous waste using water, for example, colon irrigation. However, some people think that fasting and colon purification are not mandatory for detoxification. It's a matter of personal preference eventually.

The body's key systems, such as respiratory, digestive, dermatological, urinary, and lymphatic systems, contribute to this method. If these disposal systems don't function properly, hazardous chemicals build up and overload our bodies. Thus, we can experience sluggishness and tiredness, discomfort and soreness, mental fogginess, and congestion.

Although our bodies do an excellent job of processing and removing unnecessary and unhealthy products, we can integrate many simple and natural aids into our lifestyles.

Next, we do not add to the load by ingesting "junk foods" or by exposing to smoking or applying chemical-laden skin preparations. Think of something you put in or on your body. Reduce or fully exclude alcohol, coffee, nicotine, refined sugars, and saturated fats, and don't forget the common home chemicals we use every day.

By natural detoxification, you should stop something heavily processed and conform to the easy and "close to nature" method, which will ensure that your body has far less work to do.

One of the simplest things to be vigilant about is good, clean water. Our bodies consist mostly of water, and most of us walk chronically dehydrated. How do we expect our bodies to flush all the toxins out if we do not give them enough water?

And the best is pure water. It is said that it's too late if you're thirsty. Keep ahead of the game, and make sure that you drink a good glass of water when you wake up and a little before your lunch at noon.

Again, how do we expect our bodies to work properly unless we do our part?

As our breathing rate rises and we begin to sweat through these pores in our skin, we sometimes don't think about removal methods. Instead, take the stairway—park in the parking lot more. Go for a walkout at lunchtime around the block. Sunshine is also going to do you well!

The diet, which consists mainly of raw fruit, vegetables, seeds, and nuts, also allows the body to eliminate the fiber required. This natural detox diet also provides the body with a healthy way to achieve long-term clean energy.

These are just a couple of simple things. The concept of

natural detoxification is to reduce the load of contaminants that first come into the body and then let your body work smoothly, like a fine-tuned machine.

Quick and natural detox is best for your body, and oh well! You will make every effort and feel more pep in your step! Isn't it worth that much?

CHAPTER 17

HOW TO GET A BODY CLEANSING DETOXIFICATION

It is almost impossible in our society today to prevent the accumulation of toxins in your body. Certain approaches are straightforward, some require dedication, and some can be risky. It is important to find the right body cleansing detox method for you that does more than hurt.

In the food we consume, liquids we drink, and the air we breathe, we are bombarded with chemicals. Butylparaben, benzoic acid, benzene, bentonite, BHT, BHA, and bronopol are not common names, but they may not be common harmful to foods, cosmetics, or cleansers. They are relatively common toxic substances. Perhaps worse, the alphabet includes 25 more letters.

Our bodies are doing a courageous job of removing toxins. They filter the contaminants in the kidneys and liver and then expel them by sweating and the rest of our excreta. If this natural detox system is overloaded, it contributes to toxic overload. The results can lead to breathing, digestive, and other general problems of health.

Fortunately, it is possible to help the body cleanse itself of poisons, including:

Herbal additives
Herbal wraps of the body
Plans for cleaning
Dietary changes
Saunas

Herbal supplements can be used to clean up the body, usually as tablets. They can affect your body's work by increasing the number of antioxidants, certain vitamins, and minerals. The more effective excretion of toxins can include this shift.

It becomes a challenging business to adjust your body's basic chemistry so that you are assured of a full understanding of the entire process before embarking on a journey of this nature. Your doctor can help you direct you to whatever action plan you choose, not just the Internet.

Herbal body wraps are typically a combination of clay, salt, water, and/or some other ingredients such as oils. The theory is that the salt draws water from the skin to create toxins. This normally means lying in a mixed space for up to an hour or longer. It is critical that you afterward drink plenty of fluids to replace the flushed water in your body.

Some people go to a spa or find a set program to use a tissue purification plan. Many plans include full daily schedules of enemas, beverages for purification, and liquid supplements. This series is repeated all day long.

This approach requires determination, commitment, and a carefully calculated schedule over a week or more. You must be sure that the program comes from a reputable source and is administered with enough guidance.

People also change their diets temporarily or for a long time to purify their systems—many of the toxins that we produce come from the food we consume. Processed foods include, among other things, pesticides, herbicides, and artificial hormones, but also natural products such as fruits and vegetables.

A popular foundation for detox diets is to fast, eat whole organic foods, mostly vegetables, and drink plenty of fluids, particularly water. The routine use of this washing procedure, "clean you out," should be used carefully for long periods. A balanced diet needs many vital nutrients. Any of them may be ignored if this small diet is overdone.

My preference and maybe simplest (my form of the plan) are using a detox sauna. The natural way to remove toxins is through the excretory mechanism from our bodies. Sweating is a function of the excretory mechanism under-appreciated.

The reality is that the sweating method removes an astonishingly large volume of fluids. The accumulation of toxins in sweat increases significantly through prolonged sweating, as in a sauna.

That's how many of the toxins are present in the cellular fluid. The first fluids to be sweated out are the fluid that covers the cells. The fluids in the cells are washed out by unnecessary or prolonged sweating to compensate for fluids in the cell, and the dissolved contaminants go along for the trip.

Individuals were cased when extremely high levels of a certain contaminant were exposed, and a sauna was used to detoxify them. The poison was removed in such high amounts that the particular chemical was simply left to smell.

All these methods of cleaning the body have their advantages and disadvantages and can be efficient.

Which one is the best?

Ok, since they say "the one that you will use" is the one that works best. The modern home sauna market offers such a relatively low cost, comfort, and ease of use that it is not surprising that it is the option of many families. This is much harder and much more fun than any other form. Indeed, I would say that a sauna is the only body cleaning described, even if it does not have detoxification advantages.

With pace taking over all of our lives, we are largely unaware of what is going on with our body's internal organs. Because of the rapid and easy life we live, we make things even quicker by adapting to short ways of cooking our food. Who has time to think of the food they cooked today as nutritious?

Half the time in their cooking, people use cut vegetables. These cut vegetables, as well they are packed and stored, are bound to lose at least some content of vitamins and nutrients.

Wherever you see, things are streamlined and made for busy people, and they are used to the luxury of using ready-to-cook products. They cannot know that they are on the road to potential diseases.

Here are a few good reasons why you should detox your body thoroughly:

With the quick and easy lives that we live, we are bound to have massive amounts of toxic substances in our bodies piled up. The detoxification process allows us to extract these harmful substances from our bodies that cause a lot of damage to the body organs if they build up for a long period.

Another explanation is that the body loses its normal capacity to consume nutrient content in food when packed with various kinds of toxic substances. The body thus receives inadequate doses of vitamins and minerals. Detoxification tends to reduce this.

The organ's efficiency is impaired by the accumulation of these harmful substances in our bodies and their place of accumulation. Take smoking, for example.

Toxic compounds are piled up in the lungs and cause a lot of lung damage unless they try to overcome chronic behaviors. Detoxification thus helps to eliminate harmful compounds, which are often stored in the body because of addictions.

CHAPTER 18

TOP 10 ACID-FORMING FOODS TO AVOID

What Are High Acid Foods?

High acid foods have always been a part of life. Unfortunately, these things can lead to serious health problems. Recently the connection between an acidic body status and cancer has been discovered. Much of this acid build-up comes mainly from the types of food that people consume.

A well-balanced diet will have a 75 percent /25 percent breakdown on the alkaline and acid consumption, with higher alkaline sources. The content of acid or alkaline status in any material is measured on the pH scale.

This scale runs ranges from zero to 14, with seven being the perfectly balanced median. The lower the amount, the higher the acid content. The reverse is valid for deciding how alkaline a material might be.

A high acid food is any food source that is noted to have a low pH number. Generally, most vegetation is naturally alkaline even though some acids, such as citrus, are in excess. On the other side, animal-based products are usually acidic. Animal protein, dairy products, and fats typically have a very high content of acid.

Why are high acid foods an issue?

In general, these kinds of food sources can be nutritionally very safe. A highly acidic source of food can reduce the body's pH balance over time. The oxygen content of cells can decrease, and waste materials can also build up. Over time, the formation of lactic acid and other waste materials will lead to cells transforming into cancerous tissue masses.

The higher body content of acid also doesn't work. Energy levels appear to be lower, and because of the type of food supply, higher concentrations of acid are detected; they may also be overweight. It's no secret that the same things are high in calories. Higher body acid levels are also noticed in people with poor immune resistance and low white blood cell levels.

The human body was designed to function as an alkaline being. Most human bodies function most efficiently when the body has a pH level of 7.4.

What are A Few Different Acid Foods?

The fleece of all kinds is normally acidic. In nature, even heart-healthy fish are very acidic. In general, animal protein carries a significant amount of acid intake in the average human diet. Cheese, whole milk, and similar dairy products are common elements that improve the body's acidic character.

The best way to keep your body alkaline is to consume mainly alkaline foods with little acid addition. A balanced diet could consist of an alkaline diet of 75% with an acidic disposition of 25%. If you want to elevate your pH, you have to consume more alkaline foods and probably ingest sodium bicarbonate to eliminate waste in your body and increase your pH balance.

Suggested alkaline foods include vegetables, including carrots, and fruit such as citrus fruits. Fish and fortified milk are valuable acidic foods that are moderately consumed because of their nutrients. Due to the acid content, however, they should be consumed in limited quantities.

Foods that form acid are no less than poison. All diseases originate from the acidic environment, which is produced by the consumption of acidic foods. Thus, many microorganisms target our bodies' immune systems, and it is very difficult for our vital bodies to perform their usual functions. Foods that form acid are seriously hazardous to health.

Animal flesh tops the acid map that shapes foodstuffs. Acid ash in our bodies is left in all types of meat like beef, chicken, oyster, lamb, and fish. Foods that are high in acidity cause a lot of body damage. More than 20% of the food we consume does not contain foods that form acid. The ideal alkaline ratio of 80 to 20 should always be kept in the food we have.

The category of such foods also includes dairy products and animal fats. Olive oil can also be used to cook as vegetable oil is also known as such foodstuffs. The plants belonging to this group are lentils, winter squash, and maize. Blueberries, currants, and cranberries are acidic foods as well.

Alcohols and drinks such as tea and coffee are also in this category. Also, cold beverages, cocoa, and pepper contain high acidity. You should also strive to stop as much as possible vinegar as it is acidic.

The packaged foods on the markets are all such foods, and we should try to stop them. Fresh fruit should be eaten at home and washed or cooked at all times. Cooking kills vital nutrients so that raw fruits and vegetables should always be given priority over overcooked food.

Foods that form acid are synonymous with poison. Both are going to kill you. In the acidic climate, all diseases flourish, and these foods contribute to this acidic environment. It is not only overcome or overwhelming the body's immune system by various microorganisms that attack our vital organs that it is also difficult to perform their normal functions.

All that we eat can be classified into three main categories: acidic, alkaline, and acid-based ones. Alkaline foods leave an alkaline ash in our body and help to establish an alkaline pH. On the contrary, the acidic foods tilt the pH concentrations to the acidic side.

As all body tasks are acidic, they require an alkaline atmosphere to continue to function. Oxygen and nutrients must be taken by cells and toxins removed. When an acidic environment surrounds them, they cannot do so and ultimately get sick. We ingest to produce more acid than we need in our bodies is severely harmful to health.

Animal flesh in the acidic food chart is very heavy. All meats like beef, lamb, chicken, fish, and oysters have acidic ash left in their bodies. They harm the body greatly. Acid-forming foods do not constitute more than 20 percent of our intake. The optimal ratio of alkaline acid is 80 to 20, and everything we consume should reflect this.

Animal fats and dairy-derived fats also contribute to the production of acid within us. Even vegetable petroleum is to blame. When looking for a cooking medium, you should stick to olive oil. While olives help make acid, their oil does not.

Corn, lentils, and squash in the winter are the only acidic foods. All the other foods are alkaline. Also in this group is cooked spinach. Except for cranberries, blueberries, and currants, the fruit is healthy and alkaline.

Wheat, just bread, Kamut, corn, barn wheat, macaroni, rice, noodles are all harmful and can constitute not more than 20% of our total intake. Dairy goods, such as butter, cheese, yogurt, and ice cream, are acidic and not health-friendly. Instead of natural milk, still, milk as such should be avoided and soy milk used.

Tahini, walnuts, cassava nuts, peanuts, and pecans may all cause acid and body damage. Almonds, however, are not acidic and should be tried in their diet. Sugar, maize syrup, and carob are all part of the issue, and stevia can instead be used as a sweetener.

Alcohols all help to acidify the body, and drinks such as coffee and tea. Cocoa, pepper, and cold beverages are extremely harmful. Soda thus upsets the acid/alkaline equilibrium and requires roughly 32 glasses of water to balance a glass of soda.

Vinegar is also part of the issue and should be avoided absolutely. All refined foods are acidic and fresh ingredients should be eaten and well washed and not too fried. Cooking kills nutrients, so that raw fruit and vegetables should be favored overcooked fruit.

You will take acid-forming food to the grave, so wake up and change the way you eat immediately.

Acid Reflux Foods

There are acid reflux foods to avoid if the hyperacidity condition is managed successfully. To be safe, it is important that the pH level (potential hydrogen) in the body, i.e., acid and alkaline, is balanced. Since the body tends to build up acid and become more acidic over time, an alkaline diet covering different green vegetables and fruits is essential.

Alkaline products may also include broccoli, cantaloupe, almonds, vinegar for apples, celery, dried dates, figs, lemon, lime, raisins, mangoes, melons, papaya, peanuts, algae, and watermelon. While lemon is a citrus fruit, its properties shift to high alkaline levels once ingested. Lemons are good for the acid crisis, therefore.

Acid reflux causes

Let us look at what causes acid reflux. Acid reflux (GERD) is a disease in which the stomach contents flow back into the esophagus, causing heartburn and other issues. When food is consumed, it normally moves through the stomach from the mouth, through the esophagus.

A valve made of muscle fiber, known as the lower esophageal sphincter, which closes the esophagus' stomach, prevents the re-entry of food into the esophagus of the esophagus.

This valve is often not fully developed and does not close completely. Food and stomach acid migrate back into the esophagus in these conditions. This disorder is referred to as 'acid reflux.' This can cause both acid, ulcers, and even cancer, painful symptoms, and damage to the esophagus.

Symptoms

There may be some common symptoms:

- Heartburn or chest pain.
- Heaviness or bloating sensation after eating in your stomach.
- Feeling food trapped in the esophagus.
- Nausea after eating.
- An impulse to continue burping or burping.
- Stomach pain in the upper abdomen.

These symptoms tend to get worse when someone lies down or at night.

Other signs, less common, maybe:

- Cough is recurrent.
- Swallowing trouble.
- Regeneration of food
- Hiccups
- Asthma or wheezing type signs.
- Sore throat.

These symptoms can be minimized by some simple things such as:

- Do not participate in extreme physical activity immediately after feeding.
- Nothing close around the waist

- Eating two hours or more before bedtime.
- Eat small meals at regular intervals
- Stress avoidance.
- Keep body weight under control.
- Not to burn.
- Keep the top of the body up to 45 degrees during sleep.

Acid reflux can be avoided easily by maintaining a healthy alkaline diet. Medicines or surgery may be preferred for more serious cases. Indeed, milder types of acid reflux can be effectively controlled by a healthy balanced diet and lifestyle.

Some food types cause reflux of acid. It leads to understanding what these foods are and trying to stop them. However, foods with alkaline properties such as lemons should not be confused.

Alcohol, caffeine, sugar, carbonated beverages, certain citrus fruits and juices, tomatoes, popcorn, high-fat foods, spicy foods, fatty foods, mint, onions, or fried foods are the acid reflux foods to be avoided. Sticking to an alkaline diet not only helps to control acid reflux but balances the entire body's pH for optimal health.

Find out the three basic alkalizing steps to get fitness, energy, and optimum weight instantly - quick.

Acid reflux foods are available for avoiding macaroni and cheese, spaghetti and sauce, orange juice, and mashed potatoes. Some of the above foods should be strongly avoided, but a physician or doctor should be consulted before this is achieved.

Chocolates, chocolate, cold beverages, soda drinks, and foods or fruits containing lime acid are other things to avoid at all costs. This is because they can intensify the acid levels that cause heartburn.

The severity of his condition varies from person to person, and as such, it is best to consult a doctor first before one tries to seek care from someone with the same problem.

If one wishes to start some diet for different reasons, it is best to consult a physician who can track the condition first. If the esophagus is too small, it does not work properly and makes nourishment to pass back to the stomach's throat.

Pregnant women, people with irregular eating patterns, heavy smokers, and children are mainly vulnerable to this disorder. Several suggestions have been made for the cure of this condition. They include medications, home remedies, natural cures, and herbal therapies. Real eating also plays a key role in dealing with this issue.

Eat slowly and exercise more frequently in small doses, and drink sufficient water to detoxify the system. Fried and fatty meats are the number one food to avoid. They appear to digest longer and can place more pressure on the stomach. Also, fried foods such as fries and onion rings should be avoided. You should stay away from onions and all forms of acid reflux food are to be stopped seriously.

Large food portions can contribute to acid reflux before bedtime. Large quantities of food will place great pressure on your abdominal walls at any meal. As this pressure increases, the lower esophagus valve begins weakening and can eventually open, allowing food and acid to penetrate your skin, creating an uncomfortable chest-centered burning sensation.

Coffee and alcohol- An acid recycling food to avoid

The acid reflux does not function well with caffeinated drinks and foods. Another acid reflux food to prevent involves some spices, caffeine, and citrus fruits, as these could cause acid reflux episodes. Avoid drinks proven to cause the disease.

Caffeinated beverages can increase stomach acidity. Limit your daily intake to two or fewer cups of coffee if possible. All acid reflux food is coffee and tea to avoid when it comes to acid reflux drinks list. It doesn't matter whether they're caffeinated or decayed.

Acid reflux food refined to avoid

To treat symptoms of acid reflux, it is important to include fiber in your diet. You should get enough fiber or sprinkle your food or drink with powdered fiber supplements. Fibers are made of whole grains, some fruit and vegetables, beans, nuts, and seeds. Unprocessed foods are perfect with acid reflux

An acid reflux diet to stop Gassy fruit and vegetables

Even acid reflux food for avoiding gassy fruits and vegetables. Keep away from gassy fruits and vegetables. This sadly means that certain healthier options don't form part of your food plan. Fruits and vegetables are usually alkaline and should be taken in appropriate amounts.

Another thing to avoid is tomatoes and tomato-based items. There are high acidity fruits such as citrus, grapefruits, tomatoes, and oranges. This acid content will aggravate the condition, and someone with digestive issues should avoid it.

Try to understand which kind of food helps keep the LES valve safe. Let the esophagus recover by not eating the same food as the damaged. Losing weight, exercising, properly chewing, drinking enough water, and lifting the head at night are essential. It is important to maintain a food record that causes acid reflux symptoms. Learn how to recognize symptoms quickly and get care early.

CHAPTER 19

COMMON BEGINNER DETOXIFICATION MISTAKES

The secrets of detoxification are not so hidden today. However, as with any modern and renowned medical advance, misconceptions still surround them. One is that detoxification cannot have any adverse effects on a human.

On the opposite, it is. The detoxification process is achieved using nature's power, natural components that do not include the toxic substances that could aggravate the situation.

Detoxification has its natural path, as with both natural and alternative medicines. Harmful chemicals can trigger your body to generate dramatic and very unusual signals. Though natural detoxification processes encourage a steady relief that does not cause imbalances in the body, you get effective and relaxed results.

Another misconception of detoxification includes suggesting that detoxification only benefits the colon. It's not real because we call this a myth. Yeah, detoxification focuses more on colon cleansing and cleansing the entire body system, and eliminating harmful chemicals and substances accumulated inside our bodies over time.

Worms, heavy metals, including lead and mercury, chemical accumulation, and parasites, are easily and efficiently washed out of the body using a good detoxification program.

The third myth of detoxification concerns something equal and equal to detoxification and that any improvement will, in any case, yield the same results. This is a significant mistake in detoxification since there could be several variations in detoxification programs. A very good detox program would focus not only on the colon but also on the detoxification process.

A high-quality detoxification program can also manage toxins, including heavy metals and toxins from natural sources, such as mercury from fish and other chemical toxins. It would also take on the toxins taken orally and those which our skins consume from our daily routines.

Not every detoxification program is the same, and it cannot remove toxins and other toxic substances effectively. If you plan to undergo a detoxification program, it should be perfect for you the first time.

The fourth misconception very common to detoxification states that the colon is the only organ that can accumulate toxins. This does not have an actual basis because the toxins we take from the food we eat and drink, the air we breathe is accumulated in our cells, particularly fat cells. Toxins may not only exist in our colon but also in our brain, heart, and kidneys.

They don't sit there unless we do something with them. "Any living organism, including humans, has at least one or more parasites in or on it," says Discover Magazine. The same parasites take away vital nuts and lead to the accumulation of more toxic substances in our bodies.

This implies that we are continually assaulted by substances that do not fit into our systems. The only key to detoxification is to have a sophisticated detoxification program that provides real cleaning results.

Many people understand the need to detoxify the body and thus take action. However, too often, these acts are too extreme and destructive. Below are some common mistakes to prevent during detox:

1: Too much (cold) water to drink

The use of plenty of water to flush contaminants is considered beneficial. However, when the water is cold, lymphatic drainage slows down. The detoxification mechanism is, in turn, impaired by slow lymphatic drainage because most toxins are to be flushed through the lymph system. Coldwater can also contribute to constipation, and you definitely can't get rid of any contaminants if you don't empty your bowels.

Coldwater disrupts digestion to make it worse. Indeed whatever the temperature of your drinks, you can make fewer digestive enzymes if you drink too many fluids (particularly too near to foods), and your digestion will be impaired. As a result, much fermentation can be expected in the intestines, which leads to even more toxicity.

Water can best be drunk (or slightly warm in winter) at room temperature and never during your food. Sipping hot water (alternatively with some lemon) all day long is an ideal way to melt toxins.

Drinking ginger, lemon, and honey combined first in the morning in warm water is also perfect for detoxifying. To promote lymph drainage and burn excess fat, add half (1/2) tablespoon of fenugreek powder to this mixture.

2: Too much fruit to eat

The fruit is beneficial because it includes fiber and thus facilitates daily detoxifying bowel. Furthermore, the fruit has vitamins that function as antioxidants and can contribute to the detoxification phase. However, excess fructose (fruit sugar) can be very harmful to the liver and thus a bad detox recipe.

Moreover, it can compromise the gut's health if too much fruit is mixed with other foods. In particular, you should avoid mixing fruit with milk (e.g., yogurt, cheese, etc.). When fruit is mixed with something in the intestine, it easily contributes to fermentation and increases its toxicity. Note that tomatoes are fruit as well!

Ideally, only mild fruits should be consumed alone and often between meals. Enable at least 30 minutes before and two to four hours after dinner.

3: Raw Foods

Raw foods are perfect when you're digestive system is strong. But raw food can be a murderer if your gut is poor (especially when you have IBS). Before it can be assimilated, the body must cook all the crude food you eat.

When the digestive tract is exhausted, it can only be further damaged by fresh food. To detoxify your body, you have to eat food that is light and easy to assimilate. This means for many only cooked food.

If you don't want to give up your salads, eat them for lunch instead of dinner. To make digestion and assimilation easier, add some lemon and black pepper to your salad mixtures.

4: Master Cleanse of Lemon and Salt Water Flushes

Your intestine has bacteria somewhere between 1.5 - 4.5 kg. Some of them are harmful and cause toxicity (e.g., Candida). But believe it or not, some of these small buggers aren't just good for you; they account for up to 75% of your immune system!

Without the good guys in the intestines, the bad guys will easily overtake, and toxicity will increase accordingly. The good bacteria also help you make vitamins B and K and help your immune system and digestive system.

Now everyone who did Master Lemon Cleanse also experienced the notorious salt flushes administered every morning for several days in a row. It is considered a cleansing process because it literarily breaks your intestines out by thoroughly flushing its contents with vigorous (and often painful) contractions.

I did it myself, so I speak from experience. If you opt for such flushes, you eliminate the good bacteria with the poor completely. Similar effects can be achieved in colonic irrigations, but they mostly affect the large intestine and spare the intestines.

After any drastic purge, take loads of high-quality probiotics for a long period to restore gut flora. A high-quality probiotic has billions (not millions) of bacteria per capsule and is properly preserved so that bacteria remain active.

You can also follow a strict diet for several days after purgation if you just consume light, cooked food. After purging, the intestine is exhausted, so regular food is expected to add salt to your wounds.

5: Post-Detox Regime

The most serious and the most grave mistake is frequently made immediately after the successful detox process. Very few people have the patience, experience, and autonomy to progressively implement ordinary foods. Very few people know that eating McDonald's right after you are on a strict detox regime can make you sicker than before.

If you know that you can't sustain self-discipline to break out of detox eventually, don't even bother about detox. Instead, follow a more progressive and common sense approach. Improve your eating habits slowly over time and see yourself as an investment project. Break away from imported food and take-aways.

Cut off processed grains, sugar, coffee, and alcohol. Increase your workout. This would be much more helpful to you over the long term than having a 10-day diet and then going right back to your normal waste.

CHAPTER 20

EVALUATION FOR DETOXIFICATION

Most of us certainly have already learned of detoxifying diets. A detoxification diet is a way to clean up our body systems to operate effectively and correctly, without complications or breakdowns.

Detoxification diets may help counteract stubbornness, erratic bowel movements, stomach upsets, skin problems, bloated feelings, exhaustion, extra fat, and much more. Detoxifying diets can help alleviate chronic pain.

Detoxifying diets will certainly help you lose weight in your quest. How to wonder? How? Our bodies are built to live in natural foods and substances only. Our additives are considered foreign objects by our bodies, and although they are present in us for a long time, our systems are not meant to take advantage of them.

Much of the weight stored by our bodies is linked to all the chemicals and toxins our bodies have collected. Detoxifying diet for losing weight will purify our systems and correctly distribute and use our bodies' nutrients from our food.

A weight loss detoxification diet isn't something we'd regularly do for the rest of our lives. It is just too ideal to think of losing 20 to 30 libraries by relying solely on this process.

Simultaneously, there have been instances where people claim to lose five-20 pounds of extra weight. The weight loss detoxification diet is a perfect way of purifying our system and beginning with healthy eating behaviors that eventually pave the way for better health.

How respectful would you be with being clean?

The secrets of detoxification are a gem well-guarded for quite some time. It wasn't due to its latest invention, nor was it that health professionals and physicians couldn't grasp its functions. The keys to detoxification are not obvious since it is generally rare to address it.

Your colon collects about three to four times more waste than what you excrete when you use the toilet. The normal detoxification methods and processes aren't very good, particularly when you have dinner talks.

One of the best detoxification strategies is to clean your colon of all impurities; in exchange, they rely excessively on laxatives and readily available fiber supplements. Our colon muscles have been engineered to act smoothly whenever waste is disposed of inside our bodies. When laxatives are used, the colon muscles do not have to function too hard because the waste matter within the colon is liquefied. Too many laxatives will deteriorate and weaken your colon muscles. This is because of the regular use of laxatives.

Constipation happens primarily because of the colon muscles' inability to force waste out efficiently; the muscles are no longer used to their everyday function, as it is all turned into liquid. When that happens, this bad habit becomes very unlikely to reverse.

These are couple of the reasons why detoxification strategies are kept secret. Our body system is cleansed by our digestive tract, particularly the colon, and the colon muscles are restored to routine activity.

Our dependency on laxatives and fiber supplements is now gone after the re-stimulation of colon muscles. Only think about the effect on pharmaceutical companies if the public has ever learned these detoxification secrets. The only way to get rid of our reliance on bowel medicines and fiber supplements is by detoxification.

Only think about it. The actual detoxification techniques are so dramatic and astonishing that most people assume it is too good to be true. Cleansing of the colon and our body systems is the first step towards improving our health and well-being.

Death starts at the colon and is undoubtedly real. Autopsies indicate that most people's colons are 70-80% full of too much fecal matter, which was not expelled, and the average woman in the statistics has 30 pounds more of this waste.

Many people encounter many atrocious pains that seem to have no traceable origin. These unpleasant symptoms may involve constipation, indigestion, acid reflux, heartburn, bloating, and other related issues. These unpleasant conditions are typically easy to find and can quickly and effectively be addressed by a successful detoxification program.

Other problems such as chronic fatigue, muscular pain, weak joints, headaches or migraine disease, hemorrhoids, skin problems, backaches, tooth decay, and poor breath seem to have some unrelated impact on the colon. Still, they are eventually triggered by an unclean system that certainly needs an urgent detoxification scheme.

There are certain cases where the debilitating symptoms we encounter have no relative origin and can be traced only until the cause is thoroughly discussed. It is impossible to know if the debilitating symptoms you experience come from the toxins inside your body until a full detoxification regimen is completed.

Many people are so surprised to learn that these debilitating symptoms they encounter can easily be overcome, and many wanted to discover these detox secrets sooner. In and outside of our bodies, toxins and harmful substances can affect a lot, depending on the quantity and age of these toxins and the individual's overall health. Much of the time, these toxins' effects go beyond any medicine or health specialist's ability to alleviate them.

As toxins accumulate in the human body, the thoughts can also be disturbed, and the illnesses can become lethargic and weak. This is because your body fights a largely unknown war when eye-impaired environmental toxins slowly take over without you knowing it. These toxins are what we call invisible killers. Through the air, food, and water we consume, diseases penetrate our bodies, and we don't even know they take us hostage.

If these pollutant diseases penetrate our bodies, they perturb the delicate balance needed to avoid illness and disease. Take the lead, for example; as it reaches your body, it goes straight for your bones, displacing calcium and leaving your bones fragile and broken. Mercury infects the mind where healthy neuropathic functioning is displaced.

The argument we are trying to make here is that we are all overwhelmed by this terrible threat, it's everywhere, and there's no escape. As we fight pollution issues and repair our world, we do not know that the harm has already been done.

There are things buried in this world that one day will devastate all of us, and for many years to come, our past mistakes will haunt us. The fight to save Mother Earth will continue, but we need to look at the real struggle against these pollutions.

It used to take a few years before we got to what was called a 'toxic load,' where the body was overwhelmed by so many toxins that it was pushed into tissues, organs, and fat cells. It takes a total of nine months to meet this pressure.

If you're continuously exhausted, catching cold and disease, and simply thinking well, you may be one who has reached unsafe levels. You have to act rapidly to get rid of these toxins, but you have to eradicate them every day to prevent them from occurring.

There's an elegant approach out there that can benefit you, and the stunning thing about this method is that it has zero side effects. When these chemicals are eliminated from the body, wonderful things begin to happen.

You begin to feel healthier; the organism can easily control and manage to fight disease and disease. An example of this is that a few years ago, my son was diagnosed with asthma, which helped him get rid of the illness and prevented him from becoming sick over the last two years. We forgot to sit in the doctor's office waiting to be seen, and it was truly miraculous for us.

So if you are searching for something that could change your lives, make you feel better, walk with less effort and help you recover your thoughts that you once loved when you were younger.

You might have just stumbled on what some people claim was a fountain of youth. If you look for something that could change your life and help you enjoy life entirely, then make a big deal for yourself and learn more about this wonderful tool we use.

CHAPTER 21

PRODUCTS, FOODS THAT WILL REVITALIZE YOUR BODY

It was commonly believed that colon purification could return the body to high health levels for a long time. The body accumulates toxins when waste products collect in the colon. The contaminants contained there are both environmentally friendly and nutritional.

Drugs, both recreational and prescribed, will also lead to levels of toxin. As these concentrations of toxins increase the body and lose energy, the liver's capacity has decreased, and our overall health remains subpar.

We can do a variety of things to remove these toxins.

Perform a natural colon purification system. The best way is to use natural products that work together with the normal function of the body.

Adjust your diet. This means that such foods must be avoided to reduce the number of toxins. Caffeine, nicotine, alcohol, refined sugars, and fats are among this food.

Increase workout levels. This only means adding a regular

workout into your daily life. Running 20 to 30 minutes a day is very helpful.

However, a natural colon cleaning regime is, by far, the most successful process. As mentioned above, natural products will improve the poor digestive processes experienced by a toxin-removal organ. You should also start using probiotics since you need to replenish your intestinal flora.

But what is the method of colon cleansing?

It is troubling that safe settlers usually weigh four pounds in the vicinity. Records show that an unhealthy colon can weigh up to 40 pounds in extreme cases of plaque build-up! This is significant if you know that colon cancer has the second-highest mortality rate in the United States alone.

How can you extract from your colon this dangerous plaque?

As mentioned earlier, the safest way to use natural products is to do this. You must restrict your diet to raw fruits and vegetables at the beginning. This prepares your colon for the following cleaning process. You should be checking for herbs in your intestinal tract that are known killers of parasites and worms.

Using the correct naturally occurring products containing probiotics, or beneficial bacteria as it is often called, the liver, gall, and intestines can help. Flax seeds, slippery elms, and other plants such as psyllium husk can form part of your everyday intake. The advantages of colon cleaning would be remarkably evident in around two to 3three weeks.

An increasing number of Americans use herbal supplements to improve their health instead of prescription medicines.

Natural remedies are another way to cure many of the symptoms of certain diseases.

Many herbal therapies can treat various conditions of health that can promote healthy overall well-being. For those that are exhausted or anxious, several herbs will improve your endurance. Since many have insomnia, many can need a boost.

Herbal supplements are popular for supplying some nutrients and giving you more energy and incorporating these herbal energy boosters to their diets. Herbalists claim it helps to change and revitalize the brain and body.

You will find some details on each of these additions' labels, which will help you determine what is in the packaging. The name of the supplement and the quantity of the contents are generally specified on the label. Most of these items will have a kind of disclaimer, which will indicate that the food and drug administration has not assessed the object.

The label would also include a fact sheet describing the portion size, the active ingredients, and other essential components such as amino acids. Finally, the manufacturer's name and position should be on the label. Make sure that all these items are included in the kit before buying any of these items.

Look for herbal supplements that have passed certain criteria. See which uniformity and cleanliness have been checked and free of pollutants. Many try buying single herbal products showing how much each dose of the herb has.

Do not slip down to lines that sound too good to be true. Use common sense, and if anything seems absurd, obviously the results they say will not be obtained. Also be very careful about supplements developed in other countries. Many European products are limited, but other countries do not follow the same rules as the US.

Make sure you do your homework and learn about them before taking them if you are interested in such herbal supplements. Although these items are natural, they can still be harmful to your body and should be moderated. If the side effect is unknown, consult a physician before using the medication.

The Food and Drug Administration does not require most natural health supplements to ensure protection, efficacy, or even what is included in the product. You can review all the ingredients, even with an herbal energy supplement, because you an allergic to many ingredients. Many people were admitted to the hospital for a poor response to even natural ingredients.

Some herbal supplements can fix many of a person's health problems. Before taking herbal medication, test all the ingredients, and consult a doctor if you are unsure.

Nutritional Food Supplements

For several years now, the consumption of dietary supplements has been growing. More and more people are talking and taking dietary supplements every day in today's hectic modern world. To think that it started as yet another natural herbal alternative remedy.

Today's supplements far outstrip the old herbal remedies for sophisticated processing and preparation. These nutritional supplements are also available in different types of aspects.

They are now available as tablets, capsules, liquid, teas, etc. However, a few of them are still grown and processed at home.

Why do you take dietary supplements?

Stress is one reason to take supplements, but not a clear one. Today, some people worldwide are under immense stress due to their busy everyday jobs and routine. Surely stress isn't good.

Stress decreases the body's disease resistance. This is a strong indication of stress if you are likely to get sick. Supplements are one of the easiest ways to deal with stress-related diseases. Nearly all dietary supplements boost the immune system.

As such, if you have stress-related discomfort, you certainly want to revitalize your body's immune system. You directly improve the immune system by taking dietary supplements. As such, you'll have a much stronger, attack-resistant immune system.

In general, these nutrient supplements ensure that people undertaking weight loss schemes preserve the vitamins and minerals that the body needs. Many that have a weight loss program prefer to take less food every day so that they can get enough vitamins and minerals with these supplements

Supplements also offer a balanced energy boost to fight the weight loss energy-sapping regiment. This ensures that participants in weight loss remain vigorous throughout the program.

Without vitamins, they probably will have to face a regular struggle with lethargy and have little motivation to do much.

Regardless of the reasons for using these dietary vitamins, supplements are a must in modern everyday life. If it's stress, weight loss, or just lifestyle, you'd better take supplements every day.

There are several different supplements from which to choose. You can go to a pharmacy, retail or online store and choose anyone you want. While some may be better than others in general, they all give much the same advantage.

But it's up to you to make your selection. If you practice bad eating habits, you have an increased chance that your colon will not function properly because it is obstructed!

When the colon is obstructed, contaminants build up in the bloodstream to prevent nutrient absorption. Colon cleaning is required to eliminate blockage, and it is, therefore, considered that taking herbs for the cleansing of the colon is good for one's health.

When do you have to clean up your colon?

If you encounter any of these, this may mean you already have to clean your colon, and please consult a trained person before trying:

- Fatigue
- Depression
- Indigestibility
- Retention of water
- Skin Issues
- Bad respiration
- Sleeplessness

CHAPTER 22

THE ROLE OF HERBS IN OUR BODY HEALTH, NUTRITION, AND AN EASY DIET

We all know that our diet includes vitamins, minerals, and herbs. But even though we eat well and most of us don't work for different reasons or particular requirements, we need additional supplements for our food intake. Sometimes we don't understand the importance of the maintenance, work, and health of these nutrients. That's why we forget to offer what our body needs. Let's look at our body's function of herbs.

Herbal supplements come from some plant ingredients which have been extracted naturally and prepared for particular purposes. These strong ingredients can cure the body when properly prepared and used and prevent minor and major diseases and diseases.

The disparity between herbs and medicines sometimes occurs. Through my substantial reading on this subject, I never found anyone who had a direct reply. But both plants and medicines are used for medical purposes to bring this in their best and shortest descriptive form.

For medicines, individual plant ingredients are used to generate a potent effect by chemical compounds that show biological activity, in addition to the pure value of this plant ingredient.

The same special ingredient is used with herbs (as opposed to isolated) in conjunction with other ingredients contained in the plant by nature. This synergy gives a balance and a counterbalance to the stronger ingredients, which function together with the body's natural elements.

Of course, various explanations, extensions, advantages and drawbacks, and debates on both sides of the medicine and herbal scientific role will come from here. But this is most straightforward response to explain the distinction between medicines and herbs in terms of the use and effects of either drug in our bodies.

Herbal medication is available in the following pills, tablets, syrups, extracts, teas, powders, foods, and other practical ways to provide the plants' advantages. Herbs are also used for cooking, cosmetic, medical, or decorative purposes. Different parts of different herbs, including leaves, seeds, stems, and roots, are used. They are typically used in homeopathic medicines.

Herbal medicinal products were known and used by native Egyptians, Persians, Hebrews, Romans, Chinese, American, and other nations worldwide for a decade until the early nineteenth century when modern pharmaceutical companies started isolating the individual active ingredients drug manufacturing.

In recent years, however, researchers began to look at herbal remedies again, and thus, the use of herbal medicine has gradually increased with a revived interest.

Herbal natural pharmacy is rich in substances that are helpful to different parts of the body, such as tissues, muscles, glands, and organic and biological portions of all systems in general. It includes many herbs and herbs that can be used as natural medicines to prevent, treat, and cure infections, sicknesses, and diseases.

It supplies herbs that nourish and stimulate the immune system, repairs the liver, strengthens the glandular system, regenerates damaged tissues, prevents chemotherapy side effects, etc.

Two general types of medicinal herbs are tonic and stimulant. Tonic helps preserve the sound or equilibrium between the cells, tissues, and systems of the body. Some tonic herbs activate and revitalize body functions, and others provide essential nutrients required to function correctly.

Stimulating herbs provide stronger therapeutic measures on the body's parts and structures and treat special disorders, illnesses, or diseases. Therefore, they are taken for shorter times in smaller doses than tonic herbs and should be pursued with a health professional's aid.

Herbal teas are highly beneficial when used consistently for several conditions over a long period. Hundreds of herbs and herbal blends can be practically protected and spoken about.

This goes beyond the reach of this paper; however, to offer a general understanding of the significance of adding herbs to our program for health improvement, as for any health problems, consulting with your doctor before making any substantial supplementary changes is always advisable and recommended.

10 natural herbs that will make your life easier

Many herbs are available to choose from if you consider colon cleansing. Here are the ten best choices:

Psyllium Husk - contains fiber and helps the intestines to strengthen.

Flaxseed - decreases inflammation and feeds membranes cells.

Seed fennel - refreshing the breath, improving digestion, relieving abdominal pain, and reducing gas.

Aloe Vera - natural laxative; relieves constipation and inflammation of the intestine.

Lung - purifies the blood, improves bile flow, decreases eczema, and helps liver function.

Ginger - improves the digestive system and restores your muscles and glands.

Ginseng - eliminating fatigue and detoxifying the whole body.

Green Tea - detoxifies the anti-oxidant and anti-inflammatory properties of your system.

Red clover- relaxes the lining of your digestive muscles, rids the circulation of toxins, and suppresses appetite.

The root of rhubarb - stops constipation.

By adding such herbs to your diet, you can start your way to a healthier and happier life!

If you want to start fresh and revitalize your body, pumping your body full of chemicals is the last thing to consider. Some people prefer to use supplements to detoxify the body, while others simply want a natural colon to cleanse to achieve the desired results. If you want to lose weight or just stop having colon cancer, here are excellent recipes and ingredients to make any natural cleanser great!

Although you normally assume plenty of natural colon cleaning recipes, you can be shocked by the time you check. Psyllium seeds are one of the key ingredients you need to look for in your recipes. This is a very natural and common product, used for the natural purpose of colon cleanse. You may take this ingredient directly with water or combine it with another recipe.

Water will be the main ingredient of which you will need enough. Water has been shown to help break down the toxins and waste and remove it from the system. It could be that you are dehydrated.

Try to bring a bottle of water to get the natural nutrients you need to keep your system free and safe. Many other natural herbs and fresh ingredients provide the best natural colon cleaning they can find. Make sure you do some homework to make sure you have the right ingredients and the best recipe you can find!

CHAPTER 23

MAINTAIN A HEALTHY BODY WITH AN ALKALINE DIET

Many of us have heard of the high alkaline diet. This form of diet has proven to be effective and beneficial. You need to have this diet to improve your immune system and keep your life safer.

Alkaline diets are a sort of diet that helps you to eat a lot more alkaline foods than acidic foods. The intake ratio of alkaline to acid must be 4:1. Alkaline foods offer us more benefits.

On the other hand, acidic foods are foods that we consider to be detrimental to our health. These include dried food, red meat, dairy products, and other products. Omega-6 fat foods are harmful to our wellbeing and are considered acidic. This includes maize oil, sunflower oil, and soy oil.

We know that having meat fats isn't very healthy. High cholesterol levels and blood pressure are triggered. Fats and carbohydrates are not healthy when consumed in large amounts. Carbohydrates are divided into metabolism carbohydrates. The sugar is then processed as fats when we eat foods that contain so much carbohydrate and don't get active.

Such fats are to blame for an unhealthy lifestyle. So many diseases and obesity are induced. Many westerners have severe weight gain issues. This is because they have more volatile foods in their diets.

How do we keep our bodies healthy?

Eat more new vegetables and fruit

We know that we have healthy fruits and vegetables. Some are known as alkaline food. Only handfuls aren't. In its natural state, even those fruits and vegetables that are acidic are called alkaline food. Lemons, lime, and grapefruits are among them.

Alkaline foods produce alkaline ash and neutralize acid ash within the body when metabolized by the body. A high alkaline diet is key to our wellbeing. High acidity causes our bones and other joints to weaken because acid eliminates calcium and other neutralizing nutrients. We should, therefore, have a high intake of alkaline foods of that type. If we did, we would regain our fitness.

Daily workout

Regular exercise helps a person get healthy and makes the mind and body function well. It also helps to ensure the proper supply of oxygen in our body. It also helps to digest well and encourages healthy eating habits.

Drink plenty of water

When you drink alkaline water, it's much healthier.

We can also drink plenty of water besides eating a high alkaline diet. But we need to learn it's easier to alkalize our water. We call this alkaline water. It's well known for our wellbeing.

You will agree that a diet called alkaline is not attractive. This is also known as the diet of alkaline acid or an alkaline acid diet. It is a diet that stresses the consumption of fresh fruit and vegetables.

The alkaline diet is not as daunting as the name makes it look, although it varies significantly from what most people consume. It is focused on consuming a few planes or animals processed.

The definition is very plain. You must eat foods you know are good for your health like salads and fresh leafy vegetables and avoid things that are not like alcohol, yeast, bad grains, and sugar. You must eat that is good for your health.

Research is slighter than this basic breakdown, but it's necessary to optimize the amount of alkaline fruit, vegetables, and alkaline juices and waters that you consume.

This illustrates the 80/20 division of alkaline food into acidic foods. That's the ratio you want. Don't worry if it sounds too complex, because it isn't. Some of the foods we eat are either alkaline or acidic when completely digested. Fish, cereals, meat, shellfish, poultry, salt, and milk contain acid, all of which are popular in the Western diet.

Although you should eat more alkaline foods like fresh fruits and vegetables, this is not always true. As a result, we have very alkaline blood, but with regular pH levels from 7.35 to 7.45. You should consume a diet that represents your body's pH level, and that is somewhat alkaline, and it was for our ancestors.

The main explanation for this is that most have never heard of an alkaline diet nor the body's alkaline acid balance. Still, holistic physicians and nutritionists are also advocates of this diet as this form of treatment is considered necessary to remain healthy and avoid diseases such as cancer.

Most mainstream physicians, on the other hand, don't believe or endorse the alkaline diet.

How does one want to eat alkaline? Some claim that an alkaline diet can benefit chronic diseases. There are currently a few medical studies to support this specific diet, but most of the foods it allows you to consume are nutritious foods approved by most physicians.

This diet may benefit people who don't feel well while eating a diet low in carbohydrates or high in protein. It may also support those who live stressful lives and consume too many acidic foods. For example, talking to the doctor before committing to a diet is also a good idea.

CHAPTER 24

DR. SEBI RECIPES

1. Green Raw Soup

Ingredients

2 Avocado

1 Cucumber, peel, and seed

1 Jalapeno pepper,

1 seed of yellow or red onion,

1/2 lemon juice

1-2 cups Water or veggie stock

2 cloves of garlic

1 Garlic roasted.

Coriander

1 dc. Parsley

Instructions:

Puree in the food processor cr blender all ingredients (except onions).

Apply more or less water for the desired consistency.

Garnish with sliced onions.

2. Autumn Tomato & Advocate Soup

Ingredients:

5 big, mature tomatoes
1/4 cup ground almonds
1 cup bottom cup of natural
vegetable stock with no
preservatives or chemical
additives:
1/4 spring onion
1 / 4 cup ground almonds

1 cup bottle without
preservatives or artificial
additives
¼ teaspoon of dill seed
Dash cayenne
Sea salt with cracked black
pepper to taste.

Instruction

Place the soup in a warm oven.

Generally speaking, this diet requires some fresh citrus fruits and low sugar foods, which help reduce foods high in acids, such as grain, milk, meat, sugar, alcohol, caffeine, and fungi. This effectively reduces acidic food's daily consumption to 30 percent and raises the alkaline intake to 70 percent.

3. Super Alkalizing Green Smoothie

Ingredients

1 Good Water cup: alkaline water if possible (fresh spring water is usually alkaline)
1 cup organic blueberry
2 big unripe bananas

2 handed spinach, kale, chard, or other dark green leafy seaweed-arame, kelp,
One shot of wheat-grass juice

Instructions

Mix ingredients with some ice cubes in a blender. Mix well and enjoy. A great start to your alkaline diet, this smoothie overloads your day.

4. Chickpea and Spinach

Ingredients:

1 cup of coarsely chopped onion:
1 to 1/2 dough of ginger, chopped or rubbed
1 to 1/2 tsp of olive oil or virgin coconut oil:

1 to 1/2 tsp of red curry powder:
1 19 oz. of can chickpeas, rinsed and drained

Instructions

Heat oil gently over medium heat in a large skillet.

Remove mixture of onion and curry.

Freeze for three minutes.

Remove tomatoes and chickpeas and cook for two minutes.

Mix the lettuce, water, and salt.

Cook for another minute or until wilts is spinach.

5. Avocado Soup

Ingredients

Freshly chopped basil

1/4 tsp dry mustard

1/4 tsp salt

1 10 oz pack mixed baby greens

4 kiwis, peeled and sliced in:

1/2 ripe avocado, sown, seeded, and peeled (1/2 sliced in 8 pieces, 1/2 "cubed)

1-1/2 Tbsp olive oil

2 Tbsp of raspberry vinegar

1 tsp of grated lime peel

1 Tbsp freshly chopped basil leaves Salad

Instructions

Combine the baby greens, kiwi, grapefruit, strawberries, and star fruit in a big salad bowl. Toss and mix to spread. Put on dressing. Cover with slices of avocado.

6. Very Veggie

Amount of Servings: 4

Ingredients:

4 cups of raw spinach:
4 cups of roman spinach:
2 cups of romaine cups,
chopped in red, yellow,
orange bell pepper:
2 cups of cherry tomatoes;

1 cup of chopped broccoli;
1 cup of chopped
cauliflower;
1 cup of sliced yellow
squash;

Instructions

Top this vibrant meal with a non-fat or fatty dressing of your
choice.

7. Alkaline Detox Soup

This soup is recommended when on a detox. This recipe includes a high EFA avocado. This also contains cucumber, which is famous for its purification properties. Herbs and spices, lemon, and lime can be used.

You blend and place the avocado into a soft paste. Instead, spring onions, green or red pepper, cucumber, spinach, and garlic are added. Add Bragg Liquid Amino, light vegetables, Boullion, and lemon or lime juice.

The first thing you can do is pulp the mortar and pestle in the coriander. Add chili and lime juice to a sauce. Set it aside, and then all the vegetables are chopped finely. After that, they will be steamed but not fully cooked to prevent losing the nutrients.

Then you cover the cooked stuff and place the sauce over the rice.

It's so simple but delicious. You can also fry the vegetables with steam in a vegetable bowl if there is no steamer. You can also add creams if you are adding seafood. The product quantity depends on your preference.

8 Alkaline Snack

The alkaline snack that will most certainly appeal to your palate is lemon juice asparagus.

The ingredients include asparagus leaves, spring onions, melted (avocado) oil, rubbing lemon peel, half a lemon, fresh lemon juice, and fresh thyme.

Steam onion and asparagus in the morning but stop cooking too much. Then mix in the dressing with avocado oil, lemon juice, and thyme and lemon rind. To neutralize the lemon juice a bit, apply cold-pressed extra virgin olive oil. Put the onion and the asparagus in the spring, and then wear.

These are some of the great food recipes. You're sure going to enjoy them. Alkaline dietary recipes are balanced and tasty. All of them are healthy for your body.

CONCLUSION

The late Dr. Sebi developed this controversial and strict plant-based diet. Proponents claim to reduce the risk of disease when combined with specific dietary supplements. Dr. Sebi felt mucus and acidity induced sickness.

He proposed that consuming some foods and preventing others could detoxify the body, thereby creating an alkaline environment that could decrease disease risk and effects.

Dr. Sebi's diet is not officially accepted, and there is no scientific proof that medical problems can be avoided or discussed. Plant-based diets can improve health under some circumstances, but Dr. Sebi's diet does not provide enough essential nutrients to keep your body healthy.

The diet of Dr. Sebi allows a person to eat strictly herbal food. A necrology explains his controversial health statements, including AIDS and leukemia. These and similar allegations resulted in a lawsuit in 1993, which ended with Dr. Sebi's organization's order to stop making such statements. Dr. Sebi is confirmed to have died in police custody in 2016.

Dr. Sebi felt the Western approach to disease was unsuccessful. He held that acidity and mucus, such as bacteria and viruses, induced sickness. One of the key reasons behind the diet is that illness can only survive in acidic conditions. The diet aims to maintain an alkaline condition in the body to avoid or eliminate illness.

The official website of the diet sells botanical remedies that claim to detoxify the body. Any of these remediations — called supplements for African Bio-mineral balance — are marketed at $1,500. The platform is not related to any study that supports its health benefits claims.

It states that the Declarations have not been reviewed by the Food and Drug Administration (FDA). Many behind the platform understand that they are not physicians and do not wish to substitute medical advice with material on the site.

How to follow your diet

Dr. Sebi's Nutrition Guide provides a variety of guidelines, for example:

- Eat just the foods in the guide.
- Every day, drink one gallon of natural spring water.
- Stop animal products, alcohol, and hybrid food.
- Do not use a microwave to "kill your food."
- Stop fruits that are dried and seedless.

Dr. Sebi's diet includes:

- Vegetables such as avocados, cabbage, bell peppers, and wild spices
- Fruits, including apples, bananas, dates, and oranges from Seville
- Grains of wheat, wild rice, and quinoa

- Oils from avocado, hemp seeds, coconut, and olive oils, but the diet suggests the use of the latter two in the cooking phase
- Hemp, crude sesame seed, tahini butter, and walnuts nuts and seeds
- Herbal teas including variations of chamomile, fennel, and ginger
- Agave syrup and date sugar are natural sweeteners
- Spices, cayenne and powdered algae

Best of Luck!